CROSS-BORDER CHALLENGES IN INFORMATICS WITH A FOCUS ON DISEASE SURVEILLANCE AND UTILISING BIG DATA

Studies in Health Technology and Informatics

This book series was started in 1990 to promote research conducted under the auspices of the EC programmes' Advanced Informatics in Medicine (AIM) and Biomedical and Health Research (BHR) bioengineering branch. A driving aspect of international health informatics is that telecommunication technology, rehabilitative technology, intelligent home technology and many other components are moving together and form one integrated world of information and communication media. The series has been accepted by MEDLINE/PubMed, SciVerse Scopus, EMCare, Book Citation Index – Science and Thomson Reuters' Conference Proceedings Citation Index.

Volume 197

Recently published in this series

Vol. 196. J.D. Westwood, S.W. Westwood, L. Felländer-Tsai, C.M. Fidopiastis, R.S. Haluck, R.A. Robb, S. Senger and K.G. Vosburgh (Eds.), Medicine Meets Virtual Reality 21 – NextMed/MMVR21

Vol. 195. C.W. Cryer, A Math Primer for Engineers

Vol. 194. M.-C. Beuscart-Zéphir, M. Jaspers, C. Kuziemsky, C. Nøhr and J. Aarts (Eds.), Context Sensitive Health Informatics: Human and Sociotechnical Approaches

Vol. 193. E.J.S. Hovenga and H. Grain (Eds.), Health Information Governance in a Digital Environment

Vol. 192. C.U. Lehmann, E. Ammenwerth and C. Nøhr (Eds.), MEDINFO 2013 – Proceedings of the 14th World Congress on Medical and Health Informatics

Vol. 191. B.K. Wiederhold and G. Riva (Eds.), Annual Review of Cybertherapy and Telemedicine 2013 – Positive Technology and Health Engagement for Healthy Living and Active Ageing

Vol. 190. J. Mantas and A. Hasman (Eds.), Informatics, Management and Technology in Healthcare

Vol. 189. B. Blobel, P. Pharow and L. Parv (Eds.), pHealth 2013 – Proceedings of the 10th International Conference on Wearable Micro and Nano Technologies for Personalized Health, June 26–28, 2013, Tallinn, Estonia

Vol. 188. H. Grain and L.K. Schaper (Eds.), Health Informatics: Digital Health Service Delivery – The Future Is Now! – Selected Papers from the 21st Australian National Health Informatics Conference (HIC 2013)

ISSN 0926-9630 (print)
ISSN 1879-8365 (online)

Cross-Border Challenges in Informatics with a Focus on Disease Surveillance and Utilising Big Data

Proceedings of the EFMI Special Topic Conference
27–29 April 2014
Budapest, Hungary

Edited by

Lăcrămioara Stoicu-Tivadar

Department of Automation and Applied Informatics,
University "Politehnica" Timişoara, Romania
Co-Chair Scientific Programme Committee (SPC)

Simon de Lusignan

Department of Health Care Management & Policy,
University of Surrey, United Kingdom
Co-Chair Scientific Programme Committee (SPC)

Andrej Orel

Marand d.o.o., Ljubljana, Slovenia
Editorial Committee

Rolf Engelbrecht

KMF – Koch Metschnikow Forum, Berlin, Germany
Editorial Committee

and

György Surján

National Institute for Quality- and Organizational Development
in Healthcare and Medicines – GYEMSZI, Hungary
Chair Organizing Committee, EFMI Publication Officer

IOS
Press

Amsterdam • Berlin • Tokyo • Washington, DC

ISBN 978-1-61499-388-9 (print)
ISBN 978-1-61499-389-6 (online)
Library of Congress Control Number: 2014937361

Publisher
IOS Press BV
Nieuwe Hemweg 6B
1013 BG Amsterdam
Netherlands
fax: +31 20 687 0019
e-mail: order@iospress.nl

Distributor in the USA and Canada
IOS Press, Inc.
4502 Rachael Manor Drive
Fairfax, VA 22032
USA
fax: +1 703 323 3668
e-mail: iosbooks@iospress.com

PRINTED IN THE NETHERLANDS

L. Stoicu-Tivadar et al. (Eds.)

Preface

This volume contains the proceedings of the 11-th *European Federation for Medical Informatics (EFMI, www.efmi.org) Special Topic Conference (STC)* held in Budapest, Hungary 27th–29th April 2014. The EFMI STC 2014 is an important international forum for presenting results of current scientific work in health-informatics processes, systems, and technologies.

The EFMI STC is a major scientific meeting. It brings together computer and information science, medicine, and technology. The conference provides a comprehensive overview and in-depth, first hand information on new developments, advanced systems, technologies and applications.

The EFMI STC 2014 was organised by EFMI in collaboration with the Biomedical Section of the John von Neumann Computer Society (NJSZT, further details at: http://njszt.hu/en/neumann/about-njszt). It follows previous conferences in Bucharest, Romania (2001), Nicosia, Cyprus (2002), Rome, Italy (2003), Munich, Germany (2004), Athens, Greece (2005), Timişoara, Romania (2006), Brijuni Island, Croatia (2007), London, UK (2008), Antalya, Turkey (2009), Reykjavik, Iceland (2010), Laško, Slovenia (2011), Moscow, Russia (2012), and Prague, Czech Republic (2013).

The theme of the STC 2014 is "*Cross-border challenges in informatics with a focus on disease surveillance and utilising big-data*", addressing a range of important aspects of pan-European and cross-border issues. The conference contains sections providing state of the art presentations on the following theme areas:

- Health data sharing, integration opportunities and challenges across European borders,
- Sources of data, including big data, for monitoring health and disease,
- Using routine data for epidemiological study and public health.

The EFMI Working Groups supporting the conference include "*EFMI WG PCI Primary Care Informatics*" and "*EFMI WG HIIC Health Informatics for Interregional Cooperation*".

The objective of the conference, reflected in the contents of the present volume, was to highlight health-related use of data and the use of these data for monitoring and preventing ill health and disease. They include reports about collaboration at regional, national, and international level. Achieving and maintaining cross-border interoperability of electronic health record systems implies managing the continuous process of change and adaptation of a multitude of elements within and across electronic infrastructures in neighboring countries.

The volume contains twenty-three full papers and poster extended abstracts from specialists of the field. The papers have been selected by the Scientific Program Committee (SPC) out of forty-five submissions of papers, posters, and workshop proposals sent by experts from all over Europe, Russia, Israel and South Africa. Each submission has been reviewed by three reviewers selected from a list of internationally acknowledged domain experts from all continents. The SPC members wish to express their gratitude to the reviewers for the work, which was carried out with the utmost care. All the reviewers' names are listed in the following chapter of these Proceedings.

The topics presented at EFMI STC 2014 are interdisciplinary in nature and consequently of interest to a variety of professionals: medical informatics, bioinformatics, and health informatics scientists, medical computing and technology specialists, public health, health insurance and health institutional administrators, physicians, nurses, and other allied health personnel, as well as representatives of industry and consultancy in the various health fields.

The editors wish to thank the conference patron Dr. Miklós Szócska, Minister of State for Health of the Republic of Hungary. We wish to extended our thanks to Comp-Rend Ltd. for managing the conference and the website (www.stc2014.org), to Thomas Schabetsberger for facilitating the online congress management, and to Bernd Blobel for his caring advice with these Proceedings giving the editors a big part of his vast experience in the field. Finally, we wish to thank the local organizing committee: Dr. István Kósa, István Nagy, Gergely Héja, Gabriella Merth, and Szilvia Tóth-Csuzi.

The editors would like to thank again to all of the authors for their excellent work and the reviewers for their expertise and careful review of the papers.

Lăcrămioara Stoicu-Tivadar, Simon de Lusignan, Andrej Orel,
Rolf Engelbrecht and György Surján
Editors

EFMI STC 2014
Programme Committee and Reviewers

Program Committee

Lăcrămioara Stoicu-Tivadar, Romania (co-chair)
Simon de Lusignan, United Kingdom (co-chair)
Andrej Orel, Slovenia
Rolf Engelbrecht, Germany
Mihaela Crişan-Vida, Romania
Gergely Héja, Hungary
György Surján, Hungary (head of LOC)

Reviewers

Etienne De Clercq, Belgium
Ronald Cornet, The Netherlands
Nassim Douali, France
Rolf Engelbrecht, Germany
Arie Hasman, The Netherlands
Mira Hercigonja-Szekeres, Croatia
Thomas Karopka, Germany
Lenka Lhotská, Czech republic
Christian Lovis, Switzerland
Diana Lungeanu, Romania
Simon de Lusignan, United Kingdom
John Mantas, Greece
George Mihalas, Romania
Anne Moen, Norway
Andrej Orel, Slovenia
Carlos Parra Calderon, Spain
Brigitte Séroussi, France
Lăcrămioara Stoicu-Tivadar, Romania
Vasile Stoicu-Tivadar, Romania
Patrick Weber, Switzerland

Contents

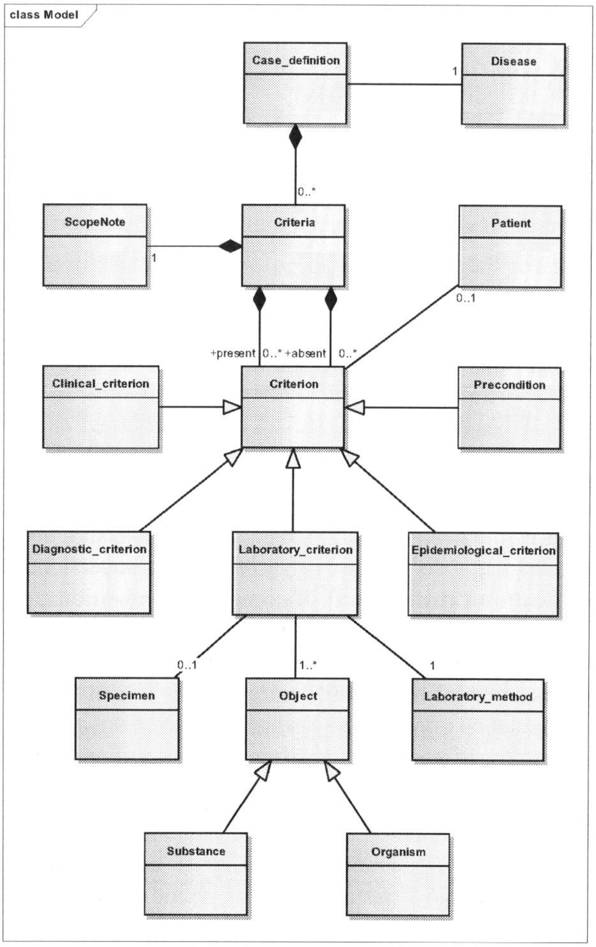

Figure 1. Class model of case definition value set

Table 1. Number of new categories in the updated value sets

Value set	Before addition	New categories	Increase
disease	809	212	26.2 %
organism	3214	28	0.9 %
public health	1930	168	8.7 %

3. Discussion and conclusions

Extracting and implementing systematic terminology from a legal text poses a number of challenges. Besides using the results for information system design and development, such an exercise can serve as a kind of quality and consistency control to the regulation itself. Such regulations should be updated and improved regularly. Besides the professional (medical, epidemiological) content the observations coming from the knowledge engineering task can further improve the general quality of the legal text. We have identified the following error types:

- **Classification errors**, e.g. "Elevated serum aminotransferase levels" mentioned as clinical criteria, being obviously a laboratory criteria,
- **Inconsistent granularity** of conditions, e.g. "Two or more health-care workers with clinical evidence of SARS in the same health-care unit and with onset of illness in the same 10-day period" versus "Laboratory exposure",
- **Seemingly nonsense criteria**, medical trivialities like "routine investigations do not suggest an alternative diagnosis" for variant CJD. There is no need to state this criterion, since this is the very process of making medical diagnoses,
- **Possible logical errors**, e.g. conditions as "A clinician's decision to treat the person with a full course of anti-tuberculosis therapy", "A case discovered post-mortem with pathological findings consistent with active tuberculosis that would have indicated anti-tuberculosis antibiotic treatment had the patient been diagnosed before dying",
- **Seemingly factual errors that might be phrasing errors**, e.g. "Demonstration of HIV by HIV p24 antigen test, including neutralisation assay" where "neutralisation assay" seems to be an p24 antigen test, "although it is a test to detect virus-neutralizing antibodies; this might be a phrasing error, if "including" was used instead of "and". "Detection of Yersinia pestis nucleic acid (F1 antigen)", where F1 antigen is a protein, not a nucleic acid.

The observed problems show that our hypothesis regarding possible improvements of the regulation is valid: there are some open issues in this text and there is room for improving the phrasing that might lead to more precise data collection and hence better understanding of infectious disease epidemiology.

Formal representation of case definitions enabling automatic classification of cases was out of scope of the project. This task would require other formalism, such as those used by rule-based decision support systems, because SKOS cannot be used to represent the assertions themselves (e.g. "Any person with at least four of the following five:"). While in principle OWL can be used to represent such assertions, the resulting ontology would be very complicated and beyond the ability of presently available inference engines to adequately handle them.

References

[1] COMMISSION IMPLEMENTING DECISION of 8 August 2012 amending Decision 2002/253/EC, laying down case definitions for reporting communicable diseases to the Community network under Decision No 2119/98/EC of the European Parliament and of the Council (notified under document C(2012) 5538), EU Commission, 2012; http://eur-lex.europa.eu/LexUriServ/LexUriServ.do?uri=OJ:L:2012:262:0001:0057:EN:PDF .

[2] L. Balkanyi, Terminology services – an example of knowledge management in public health, *Euro Surveill,* **12**(22) (2007), 3211.

[3] JJ Cimino, Desiderata for Controlled Medical Vocabularies in the Twenty-First Century, *Methods Inf Med* **37** (1998) 394-403; http://www.eurosurveillance.org/ViewArticle.aspx?ArticleId=3211.

[4] http://www.cdc.gov/phin/tools/PHINvads/ .

[5] S. Schulz, M. Boeker; H. Stenzhorn; J. Niggemann, Granularity Issues in the Alignment of Upper Ontologies, *Methods Inf Med* **48** (2009), 184–189.

[6] http://www.w3.org/TR/owl-features/.

[7] http://www.w3.org/2004/02/skos/.

[8] http://www.w3.org/TR/soap/.

[9] http://www.w3.org/TR/sparql11-overview/.

Cross-Border Challenges in Informatics with a Focus on Disease Surveillance and Utilising Big Data
L. Stoicu-Tivadar et al. (Eds.)

doi:10.3233/978-1-61499-389-6-9

Arranging ISO 13606 Archetypes into a Knowledge Base Using UML Connectors

Georgy KOPANITSA[a,b]
[a] *Institute Cybernetic Center, Tomsk Polytechnic University, Lenina 30, Tomsk, Russia*
[b] *Tomsk State University for Architecture and Building, Tomsk, Russia*

Abstract. To enable the efficient reuse of standard based medical data we propose to develop a higher-level information model that will complement the archetype model of ISO 13606. This model will make use of the relationships that are specified in UML to connect medical archetypes into a knowledge base within a repository. UML connectors were analysed for their ability to be applied in the implementation of a higher-level model that will establish relationships between archetypes. An information model was developed using XML Schema notation. The model allows linking different archetypes of one repository into a knowledge base. Presently it supports several relationships and will be advanced in future.

Keywords. Archetype, UML, Knowledge base

Introduction

Many of modern electronic health record (EHR) standards make use of the dual model architecture (i.e. ISO 13606). However, the impact of such standards is biased by the limited availability of tools that facilitate their usage and practical implementation.

The semantic of archetype data fields can be defined by linking these fields to the registers through an "ontology section" [8]. However, a generally accepted method to semantically connect different data fields or archetypes is still missing and it cannot be resolved within the Archetype model of ISO 13606. Development of a higher level model that will enable semantic linking of archetypes and certain archetype data fields within a repository can advance the application of archetype based EHR systems and facilitate for example decision support [3] or medical data visualization [5] where the context of knowledge is very important. This can be further enhanced with semantics if the archetype is linked to knowledge representations, that might, for example, enable the system to act on the information directly e.g., by triggering an alert or notification if the value contained in the Blood test instance is above normal reference suggest some action or provide other existing information. The system that receives an instance of the Blood Test observation should be also able to deliver it to a specialist, who will proceed with its assessment. Archetypes connected to business process stages will allow semantic interoperability on the process level. Classification and categorization of archetypes will reduce the entropy of knowledge.

Archetypes are defined by Archetype Definition Language (ADL) [6] that currently supports neither inference nor rules to form a knowledge base. One approach to connect archetypes into a knowledge base is the semantic web [1]. Semantic web methods of domain description may be redundant and not specific for the limited applications that use archetype medical data now.

Several methods of archetypes' transformation were developed to transform ADL archetypes to XML [10]. This allows processing of archetypes and archetype medical data and facilitates the development of higher-level models to organize archetypes into knowledge bases. To develop the information model it is necessary to define the relationships between archetypes that the model will support.

1. Materials and methods

To develop an information model and a method to connect archetypes we analysed the existing connectors' types that are used to link domain concepts. Existing UML connectors' types were analysed to find out which of them can be applied to connect different archetypes or archetype data fields and to set up the semantically meaningful relations. ISO 13606 archetype model allows definition of different relationships between archetypes connection. The structure of the ISO 13606 archetype model was studied to find out which relationships are already implemented in the model and which are missing. The examples of weaknesses and advantages of ISO 13606 models were studied and presented in the paper. Some of UML connectors [4] were implemented in the model. XML Schema approach [7] was used to specify the information model. A web-application was developed to prove the concept and test the feasibility of the developed approach. The "Association" connector was implemented to bind [value]-[Normal interval] association for laboratory results archetypes. The application was implemented in Microsoft Visual Studio using asp.net and XSL templates that process XML visual medical concept files to present EHR content to users.

2. Results

2.1. UML Connectors analysis

The following UML connectors' [4] were analysed for the possibility to be applied to organize an archetype based knowledge base:

- **Abstraction**. An abstraction relationship is a dependency between model elements that represent the same concept at different levels of abstraction or from different viewpoints. One can add abstraction relationships to a model in several diagrams, including use case, class, and component diagrams. Archetypes of one type i.e. blood test may be attributed to a different level of abstraction depending on the requirements of a certain specialist. These different abstraction level archetypes must be distinguished within a repository.
- **Aggregation**. An aggregation relationship depicts a classifier as a part of, or as a subordinate to, another classifier. This is already implemented in the ISO 13606 archetype model. Archetypes are extensible formal constraint

definitions of object structures. In common with object model classes, they can be specialized, as well as composed (i.e. aggregated). An archetype may have a container for another archetype. This can be used to define complex medical documents that consist of several concepts. However, the model implemented as including of one archetype into another while modelling and does not imply consistency if one of the archetypes is changed later.

- **Composition.** A composition relationship represents a whole–part relationship and is a type of aggregation. A composition relationship specifies that the lifetime of the part classifier is dependent on the lifetime of the whole classifier. In archetype model there exists a composition type of relationship. This is used to form whole Compositions in the EHR, e.g. for "discharge summary", "antenatal exam" and so on. However, this corresponds to the aggregation connector in UML.
- **Association**. An association relationship is a structural relationship between two model elements that shows that objects of one classifier (actor, use case, class and interface) can connect and can navigate to objects of another classifier. This is a very important relationship for medical concepts. There exist several types of associations used on the daily basis by the doctors and cannot be implemented within the archetype model of ISO 13606. For example [value]-[Normal Interval] or [Secondary diagnosis]-[Primary diagnosis] especially when the relationship is one to many.
- **Dependency**. A dependency relationship indicates that changes to a one-model element (the supplier or independent model element) can cause changes in another model element (the client or dependent model element). The supplier model element is independent because a change in the client does not affect it. The client model element depends on the supplier because a change to the supplier affects the client.
- **Generalization**. A generalization relationship indicates that a specialized (child) model element is based on a general (parent) model element. Although the parent model element can have one or more children, and any child model element can have one or more parents, typically a single parent has multiple children. Generalization is used in several archetype modelling tools e.g. LinkEHR [6]. One generic archetype can be specialized by adding specific names and values to the generic archetype. For example, a generic laboratory test archetype becomes a basis for a Blood sugar archetype.
- **Realization**. A realization relationship exists between two model elements when one of them must realize, or implement, the behaviour that the other specifies. The openEHR Template model implements this relationship where a user can specify localization properties of an archetype. For example, reference interval, data fields names, language properties and so on. However, there exist no mechanism to maintain consistency of the [archetype]-[template] relationship when the archetype is changed.

A possible archetype repository is presented in Figure 1. The proposed UML connectors connect archetypes.

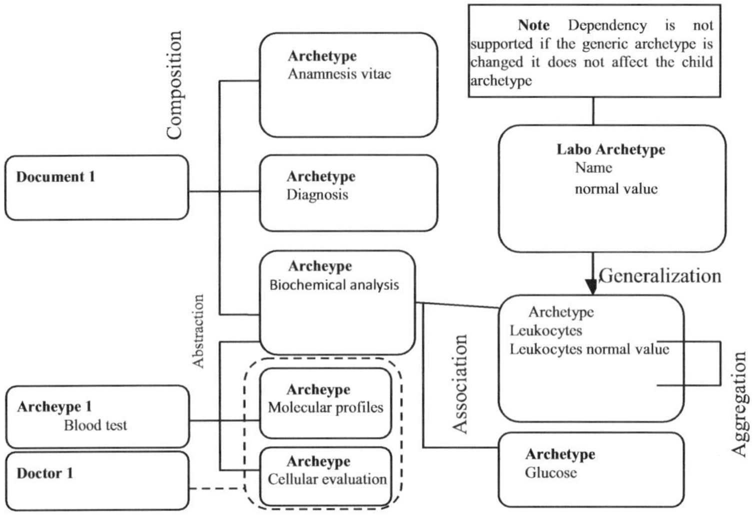

Figure 1. Application of UML connectors in an archetype repository

To demonstrate how the archetypes can be connected within a repository we can have a look at a group of archetypes for Blood tests (Figure 1.). There exist several abstractions for a blood test: Cellular test, Molecular profiles and Biochemical analysis. Archetypes can be combined to fulfil different needs. For example, each doctor can use his/her own set of archetypes, or archetypes with different level of abstraction.

2.2. Model Implementation

An information model that allows building a knowledge base was developed considering the archetype model in form of XML schema to ensure a full compatibility. Each information model entity (ME) is stored as XML file, which can be generated manually or partially automatically. An instance is logically divided into two main sections: metadata and medical content. The data fields are derived from different archetypes and combined into groups, which allow specifying the user context for each element. This allows not only connecting different archetype and archetype data fields but enables more specified description of each medical document. The developed information model is based on the archetype model of ISO 13606. The archetypes and information model instances that contain relationships between archetypes and data fields are placed on the instance level. On the data level ME files with specified content and properties are associated with corresponding medical data files.

2.3. Archetype set

In the ByMedConnect dataset, an archetype of laboratory results is represented as a set of archetypes of a similar structure. Each archetype contains one ELEMENT of type Physical Quantity (PQ) consisting of a value and a unit, one ELEMENT of type PQ interval that contains the reference interval for the measured parameter and one ELEMENT of type DATE for the date of measurement. The content of the blood test report is specified in the content section of a ME and consists of a set of elements, each referring to the corresponding archetype.

3. Discussion

Connecting archetypes within a domain model will expand the application of archetype based electronic health records. The methods to connect archetypes that are available in the ISO 13606 archetype model are not sufficient and consistent. This can be advanced by implementing a higher-level information model that supports at least the relationships that are defined in UML. The information model complementing the archetype layer must be able to provide different semantic for connectors. For example, "Association" connector may have different meanings such as [value]-[normal interval], [primary diagnosis-secondary diagnosis]. Modification of existing UML connectors in order to apply different logical mechanisms, e.g. fuzzy logic [9] and modal logic [2] will enable expressing knowledge more explicitly. Figure 1 shows the hierarchy of concepts; however, relationships between concepts of one level can exist. These relationships can be even more complex. For example, the directed association that means Results of the Blood test 1 lead to the Diagnosis 1 that leads to Medication 1.

4. Conclusion

The UML connectors were analysed for their ability to be applied in the implementation of a higher-level model that will establish relationships between archetypes. An information model was developed using XML Schema notation. The model allows linking different archetypes of one repository into a knowledge base. Presently it supports several relationships and will be advanced in future. The introduced information model allows semantic connection of different archetypes or archetype data fields. The implemented web-application shows a high potential of the approach. The relationships are now static. Further research will advance the model to enable dynamic definition of the relationships and inference rules.

References

[1] M. Arg, #252, e. Casteleiro, and J.J.D. Diz, Clinical practice guidelines: A case study of combining OWL-S, OWL, and SWRL, *Know.-Based Syst.* **21** (2008), 247-255.

[2] J. Feldman, Symbolic representation of probabilistic worlds, *Cognition* **123** (2012), 61-83.

[3] S. Garde, R. Chen, H. Leslie, T. Beale, I. McNicoll, and S. Heard, Archetype-based knowledge management for semantic interoperability of electronic health records, *Stud Health Technol Inform* **150** (2009), 1007-1011.

[4] IBM, Designing a software application using models, in, 2005.

[5] G. Kopanitsa, Standard based multiclient medical data visualization, *Stud Health Technol Inform* **180** (2012), 199-203.

[6] J.A. Maldonado, D. Moner, D. Bosca, J.T. Fernandez-Breis, C. Angulo, and M. Robles, LinkEHR-Ed: a multi-reference model archetype editor based on formal semantics, *Int J Med Inform* **78** (2009), 559-570.

[7] C. Martinez-Costa, M. Menarguez-Tortosa, J.T. Fernandez-Breis, and J.A. Maldonado, A model-driven approach for representing clinical archetypes for Semantic Web environments, *J Biomed Inform* **42** (2009), 150-164.

[8] M. Menarguez-Tortosa, C. Martinez-Costa, and J.T. Fernandez-Breis, A generative tool for building health applications driven by ISO 13606 archetypes, *J Med Syst* **36** (2012), 3063-3075.

[9] B. Prados-Suarez, C. Molina, C. Pena Yanez, and M. Prados de Reyes, Contextualized access to electronical health records in cardiology, *IEEE Trans Inf Technol Biomed* **16** (2012), 401-412.

[10] C. Rinner, S. Janzek-Hawlat, S. Sibinovic, and G. Duftschmid, Semantic validation of standard-based electronic health record documents with W3C XML schema, *Methods Inf Med* **49** (2010), 271-280.

Cross-Border Challenges in Informatics with a Focus on Disease Surveillance and Utilising Big Data
L. Stoicu-Tivadar et al. (Eds.)

doi:10.3233/978-1-61499-389-6-15

Ontologies to capture Adverse Events Following Immunisation (AEFI) from real world health data

Harshana LIYANAGE[a] and Simon de LUSIGNAN[a,1]
[a] *Department of Health Care Management & Policy, University of Surrey, UK*

Abstract. Immunisation is an important part of health care and adverse events following immunisation (AEFI) are relatively rare. AEFI can be detected through long term follow up of a cohort or from looking for signals from real world, routine data; from different health systems using a variety of clinical coding systems. Mapping these is a challenging aspect of integrating data across borders. Ontological representations of clinical concepts provide a method to map similar concepts, in this case AEFI across different coding systems. We describe a method using ontologies to be flag definite, probable or possible cases. We use Guillain-Barre syndrome (GBS) as an AEFI to illustrate this method, and the Brighton collaboration's case definition of GBS as the gold standard. Our method can be used to flag definite, probable or possible cases of GBS. Whilst there has been much research into the use of ontologies in immunisation these have focussed on database interrogation; where ours looks to identify varying signal strength.

Keywords. Biomedical Ontologies, Immunisation, Drug-Related Side Effects, Adverse Reactions, Computerized Medical Records Systems.

Introduction

Monitoring burden of vaccine preventable disease and vaccines' benefits and risk are essential elements of modern public health surveillance. Investigators are moving towards using "big data" [1]. International surveillance is likely to become more important with increased globalisation [2]. Building a common data model is important for international surveillance [3]. However, we also need automated methods that "understand" the semantics of these data [4]; ontologies formally define the semantic relationships between data items and offer the allure of enabling machine processing [5, 6].

Detection of Adverse Events Following Immunization (AEFIs) is vital if we are to quantify the benefits of vaccination. The Vaccine Adverse Event Reporting System (VAERS) is an example of a national passive surveillance method used for detecting adverse events in USA. VAERS allows direct reporting by members of the public and utilised automated methods for classifying adverse events reported to it [7]. However, such reporting systems vary between countries, collecting data in non-standard ways.

[1] Corresponding Author.

Vaccine informatics focuses on development and use of bioinformatics methods during preclinical, clinical and post-licensing stages of vaccine development and deployment [8]. This branch of informatics has largely focussed on the digitalisation of a well regulated process and ensuring complete datasets are collected and extracted from data sources. Whilst useful, we propose a much more agile approach.

The Brighton Collaboration has developed case definitions required to define AEFI; these include Guillain-Barre syndrome (GBS) [9]. GBS is rare, and very large datasets are needed to detect it [10]; a further challenge is that GBS is a clinically heterogeneous disorder. We use GBS as an AEFI to illustrate our method, and the Brighton collaboration's definition of GBS as the gold standard (Table 1). Our ontology might be used to detect the signals associated with definite or possible cases of GBS.

Table 1. Brighton Collaboration Guillain-Barré syndrome (GBS) case definition (CSF=cerebrospinal fluid)

Diagnostic certainty	Clinical criteria
Level 1	Bilateral and flaccid weakness of the limbs *and* Decreased or absent deep tendon reflexes in weak limbs *and* Monophasic illness pattern, with interval between onset and nadir of weakness between 12 hours and 28 days, and subsequent clinical plateau *and* Electrophysiologic findings consistent with GBS *and* Cytoalbuminologic dissociation (ie, elevation of CSF protein level above laboratory normal value, and CSF total white cell count < 50 cells/µL) *and* Absence of an identified alternative diagnosis for weakness
Level 2	Bilateral and flaccid weakness of the limbs *and* Decreased or absent deep tendon reflexes in weak limbs *and* Monophasic illness pattern, with interval between onset and nadir of weakness between 12 hours and 28 days, and subsequent clinical plateau *and* CSF total white cell count <50 cells/µL (with or without CSF protein elevation above laboratory reference range) or, if CSF not collected or results not available, electrophysiologic studies consistent with GBS *and* Absence of identified alternative diagnosis for weakness
Level 3	Bilateral and flaccid weakness of the limbs *and* Decreased or absent deep tendon reflexes in weak limbs *and* Monophasic illness pattern, with interval between onset and nadir of weakness between 12 hours and 28 days, and subsequent clinical plateau *and* Absence of identified alternative diagnosis for weakness
Level 4a	GBS based on a clear statement from a treating neurologist that GBS is the diagnosis being present in the medical record and there being no contradictory information

1. Vaccine related ontology development

Vaccination programmes are generally implemented in a global scale; while data related to vaccine coverage, benefits and risks are generated and managed at national level. This introduces a diversity of data, which is a challenge for global vaccination monitoring [11]. Ontologies developed to detect AEFI must cope with this complexity.

Vaccine Ontology (VO) is a community based biomedical ontology in this domain. It contains more than 5000 vaccine-specific ontological terms [12]. The introduction of the Vaccine Ontology has been followed by efforts to develop ontologies to conceptualise adverse events. Ontology of Adverse Events (OAE) and Ontology of Vaccine Adverse Events (OVAE), an extension of OAE, has been developed to formally represent and analyse AEFI [13, 14]. The Adverse Event Reporting Ontology (AERO) has been introduced to standardise reporting of AEFI [15]. VO has largely been used to ensure the completeness of data capture about AEFI rather than, as we propose to systematically identify cases from clinical databases. They take little account about the granularity of the coding system, the nature of data recording, including free-text records when searching for signals of possible AEFI [6].

2. An AEFI ontology to detect GBS signals across multiple coding systems

We propose an ontology, which will be useful for formally integrating adverse event data from computerised medical records (CMR). This process takes into account the degree of specificity with which the clinical concept can be represented within the extractable CMR data; at present largely coded data [7]. The ontology will detect signals of varying specificity and sensitivity depending on the data available. We can classify the outputs as having complete, partial or no clear mapping (Table 2).

Table 2. Class of mapping possible from the ontology

Class	Mapping	Interpretation
Class 0	No clear mapping	Possible case
Class 1-3	Partial mapping	Possible/Probable case
Class 4	Complete mapping	Definite case

Class 0 will indicate no clear mapping but one or more possible symptoms or data suggestive of a *possible case* are present. Class 1 will be given when there is a diagnosis or a compatible diagnosis only, there are different codes available in the common coding systems used (Table 3).

Table 3. Representation of GBS in different coding systems

Clinical Concept	Read Code	ICD9	ICD10	ICPC
Guillain-Barré syndrome	F370.00,F370000, F370100	357.0	G61.0	N94.1

Class 2 will be assigned when there is additional supporting administrative evidence (e.g. period of admission); Class 3 will be given if the supporting clinical evidence is present. (e.g. immunoglobulin therapy) which is part of the Brighton case definition. Finally, Class 4 is a *definite case* with all aspects of mapping complete. We may be able to compare reported levels of partially mapped with completely mapped.

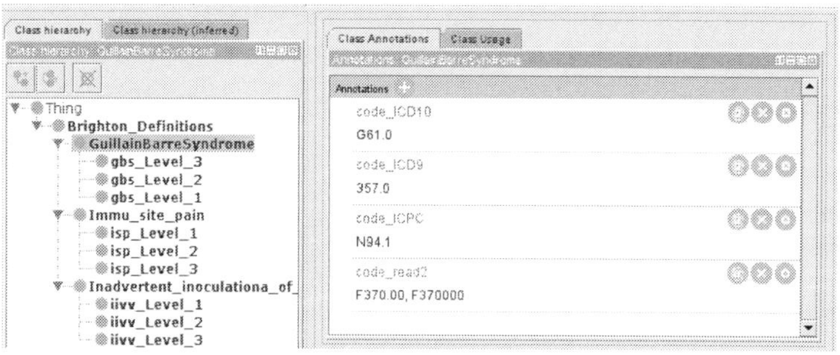

Figure 1. Representation codes for GBS in multiple coding systems

The proposed ontology has been developed (Figure 1.) using the ontology modelling tool, Protégé (http://protege.stanford.edu) [16]. The semantics of the ontology has been described according to the OWL (Web Ontology Language) specification by the W3 Consortium [17].

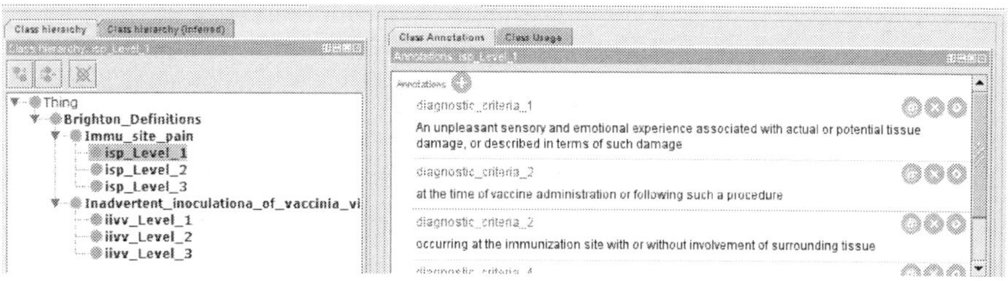

Figure 2. Representation of Brighton collaboration case definitions as ontology

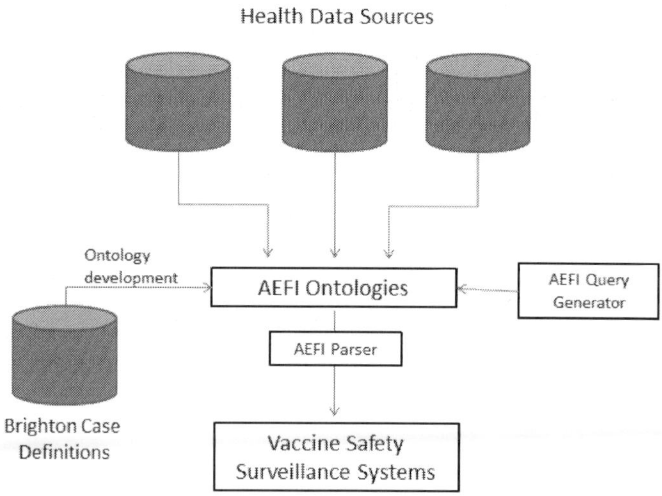

Figure 3. Parsing/extracting data from multiple coding systems using AEFI ontologies

An AEFI mapping ontology has been developed based on Brighton Case Definitions for adverse events (Figure 2). This supports annotating code from multiple coding systems. Annotated AEFI ontologies can then be used for generating queries for extracting AEFI related data from various health data sources; the associated AEFI parser can be used to parse the data and analyse a health data set (Figure 3).

3. Conclusion

Ontologies can be constructed that enable the consistent and reliable identification of AEFI, where there is both a complete set of coded data that map to a defined AEFI and the sematic relationships. The ontology will also identify possible and probable cases, which cannot be directly mapped to AEFI, but can be investigated further. Developing ontologies that define the relationship between clinical concept and coded health data is a small step towards the automated detection of AEFI from heterogeneous data sources.

References

[1] S.I. Hay, D.B. George, C.L. Moyes, J.S. Brownstein, Big data opportunities for global infectious disease surveillance, *PLoS Med.* **10**(4) (2013), e1001413.

[2] P. Kramarz, P.L. Lopalco, E. Huitric, L. Pastore Celentano, Vaccine-preventable diseases: the role of the European Centre for Disease Prevention and Control, *Clin Microbiol Infect.* (2013).

[3] Eurosurveillance editorial team. ECDC in collaboration with the VAESCO consortium to develop a complementary tool for vaccine safety monitoring in Europe. *Euro Surveill.* **14**(39) (2009).

[4] Seth Grimes, Unstructured Data and the 80 Percent Rule: Investigating the 80%, Clarabridge, Bridgepoints, (2008) Q3.

[5] H. Liyanage, S.T. Liaw, C. Kuziemsky, S. de Lusignan, Ontologies to improve chronic disease management research and quality improvement studies - a conceptual framework, *Stud Health Technol Inform* **192** (2013), 180-184.

[6] H. Liyanage et al., The Evidence-base for Using Ontologies and Semantic Integration Methodologies to Support Integrated Chronic Disease Management in Primary and Ambulatory Care: Realist Review, Contribution of the IMIA Primary Health Care Informatics WG, *Yearb Med Inform.* **8**(1) (2013), 147-154.

[7] T. Botsis, E.J. Woo, R. Ball, Application of information retrieval approaches to case classification in the vaccine adverse event reporting system, *Drug Saf.* **36**(7) (2013), 573-82.

[8] Y. He, R. Rappuoli, A.S. De Groot, R.T. Chen, Emerging vaccine informatics, *J Biomed Biotechnol.* 2010:218590 (2013).

[9] J.J. Sejvar, K.S. Kohl, J. Gidudu et al., Brighton Collaboration GBS Working Group. Guillain-Barré syndrome and Fisher syndrome: case definitions and guidelines for collection, *Vaccine* **29**(3) (2011), 599-612.

[10] C. Fokke et al..Diagnosis of Guillain-Barre syndrome and validation of Brighton criteria, *Brain* **137**(Pt 1) (2014), 33-43.

[11] P. L. Lopalco, P. Carrillo Santisteve, Actual immunization coverage throughout Europe: are existing data sufficient?, *Clin Microbiol Infect.* doi: 10.1111/1469-0691.12430 (2013).

[12] Y. He, VO: Vaccine Ontology, *The 1st International Conference on Biomedical Ontology (ICBO 2009)* (2009).

[13] Y. He, Z. Xiang, S. Sarntivijai, L. Toldo, W. Ceusters, AEO: a realism-based biomedical ontology for the representation of adverse events. Adverse Event Representation Workshop, *International Conference on Biomedical Ontologies (ICBO)*, July 26–30, 2011. NY: University at Buffalo (2011), 309-315.

[14] E. Marcos, B. Zhao, Y. He, The Ontology of Vaccine Adverse Events (OVAE) and its usage in representing and analyzing adverse events, *J Biomed Semantics* **4**(1):40 (2013).

[15] M. Courtot, R.R. Brinkman, Towards an Adverse Event Reporting Ontology. Adverse Event Representation Workshop, *International Conference on Biomedical Ontologies (ICBO),* July 26–30, 2011. NY: University at Buffalo (2011).

[16] H. Knublauch et al., The Protégé OWL Experience, Workshop on OWL: Experiences and Directions, *Fourth International Semantic Web Conference (ISWC2005),* Galway, Ireland.

[17] D.L. McGuinness, F. Van Harmelen, OWL web ontology language overview. W3C recommendation.**10** (2004):10.

Cross-Border Challenges in Informatics with a Focus on Disease Surveillance and Utilising Big Data
L. Stoicu-Tivadar et al. (Eds.)

doi:10.3233/978-1-61499-389-6-21

Comparison of Clinical Practice Guidelines from a Knowledge Modelling Perspective: a Case Study with the Management of Hypertension

Alexandre GALOPIN [a,b,c,d,1], Jacques BOUAUD [b,c,d,e], Suzanne PEREIRA[a] and Brigitte SÉROUSSI [b,c,d,f]
[a] *Vidal, Issy-les-Moulineaux, France*
[b] *INSERM, U1142, LIMICS, Paris, France*
[c] *Sorbonne Universités, UPMC Université Paris 06, UMR_S 1142, LIMICS, Paris, France*
[d] *Université Paris 13, Sorbonne Paris Cité, LIMICS, (UMR_S 1142), Bobigny, France*
[e] *AP-HP, DRCD, Paris, France*
[f] *AP-HP, Hôpital Tenon, DSP, Paris, France; APREC, Paris, France*

Abstract. Hypertension, as a cardiovascular risk factor, is a public health issue for which many clinical practice guidelines (CPGs) are published. In order to build the knowledge base of a clinical decision support system for the management of hypertension, we analysed three contemporary (2013) CPGs written in French on hypertension in a knowledge modelling perspective. We developed a semi-automated method using natural language processing called term extraction. Relevant candidate terms have been mapped to medical concepts to produce the conceptual coverage of each CPG. Only 53% of the 88 identified concepts were shared by the three guidelines. While sharing concepts does not warrantee that CPGs contents are similar, this also emphasizes guideline specificities. Such specificities could enrich the knowledge base of decision support systems by broadening their scope.

Keywords. Practice guidelines as topic, Hypertension, Medication therapy management, Natural language processing, Clinical decision support

Introduction

Clinical Practice Guidelines (CPGs) are developed by national health agencies, *e.g.* *Haute Autorité de Santé* (HAS) in France, or health professional societies, to improve the quality of clinical care and to reduce inappropriate variations. CPGs are usually elaborated as textual documents, sometimes including tables and graphics, organized as a set of theoretical clinical situations for which evidence-based therapeutic recommendations are provided. Many studies have shown that the sole dissemination of narrative CPGs has nearly no impact on physician behaviour. On the opposite,

[1] Corresponding Author.

numerous reviews suggest that clinical decision support systems (CDSSs) are appropriate tools to promote the use of CPGs [1].

Cardiovascular disease is the leading cause of preventable deaths worldwide. The majority of cardiovascular disease is due to risk factors that could be controlled, treated or modified. Numerous CDSSs [2] have been developed to support the management of one risk factor. More ambitious, our objective is to build a CDSS for the global management of the three main risks, *i.e.* hypertension, cholesterol and diabetes. The first step is to formalize corresponding CPGs and to translate these narrative documents into a computer-interpretable format. We started the work with hypertension. Because the last version of French CPGs on the management of hypertension provided by the HAS dates back to 2005, we first conducted a literature search to identify the best up to date CPGs to be considered as knowledge resources for the CDSS.

We selected three CPGs published in French in 2013: *(i)* CPGs developed by the Vidal company [3], called Vidal-Recos HTA (VR-HTA), *(ii)* CPGs developed by the French society of hypertension [4] or *Société Française d'HyperTension Artérielle* (SFHTA), and *(iii)* the annual evidence-based recommendations developed by the Canadian Hypertension Education Program (CHEP) [5]. CPGs written in English were not considered for this preliminary work to avoid multilingualism issues. Moreover, latest NICE guidelines are from 2011, the European Society of Hypertension guidance was published in late 2013, and JNC8 was not yet published.

Although published the same year on the same topic, these three CPGs looked quite different in length, structure, and content. Indeed, guideline authors provide interpretation of the available evidence and include their expertise to formulate the recommendations. Previous studies reported inconsistencies between CPGs developed on the same topic. For instance, Georg et al [6] analysed four CPGs published between 2003 and 2006 on the management of hypertension and identified various types of differences among which the selection of bibliographic references, the interpretation of these references, and the actual formulation of recommendations. It was thus difficult to objectively choose which CPGs were the most appropriate.

The aim of this work is to compare VR-HTA, SFHTA and CHEP. This involves structuring CPGs content. In the DeGeL method [7], CPGs are manually structured (first converted into semantically semi-structured text and semi-formal language by a medical expert). Other approaches involve the use of heuristic-based information retrieval [8]. We used natural language processing techniques, *i.e.* term extraction, to identify relevant terms from the narrative texts. These terms were then mapped to relevant medical concepts to produce the conceptual coverage of each CPG. Comparing CPGs was performed through the comparison of their conceptual coverage.

1. Material and Method

Term extraction has been and still is a challenge for anyone interested in domain-specific information retrieval. Approaches to automatic term extraction usually make use of linguistic processors (part of speech tagging, phrase chunking) to extract terminological candidates, *i.e.* syntactically plausible terminological noun phrases. Terminological entries are then filtered from the candidate list using statistical and machine learning methods. Once filtered, because of their low ambiguity and high specificity, these terms are useful for conceptualizing a knowledge domain or for supporting the creation of a domain ontology. Numerous software tools dedicated to term extraction have been developed. TermoStat [9] is an online terminology extractor able to extract simple as well as complex terms, from whole sentences as well as isolated words. As compared to other tools, TermoStat adds another step of statistical comparison with a reference corpus made of a large heterogeneous collection of textual documents. A score is given to each candidate terms, calculated from its relative frequency. TermoStat covers several languages, including French.

If the target users of the three selected CPGs were general practitioners, authors of CPGs, although experts in the content topic area were different. VR-HTA are developed by Vidal, a well-known French company specialized in the provision of "gold-standard" drug information, recently engaged in the authoring, development and integration of expert-based recommendations synthesized from different already published CPGs. VR-HTA are drug-centred and emphasize drug contraindications and interactions. VR-HTA guidelines are 19 pages long, and include five references. SFHTA guidelines are developed as a synthetic memento. They are voluntarily very short (4 pages, 40 scientific publications) and only explore general cases of hypertension. CHEP guidelines describe all the aspects of hypertension management and are yearly updated. The full recommendation is 35 pages long.

The method we developed to identify relevant medical concepts and produce the conceptual coverage of each CPGs relies on five different steps:

1. *CPGs pre-processing.* Narrative CPGs need to be pre-processed to allow computer analysis. Every structured element (tables, images and graphics) has been converted into raw text to avoid incorrect flattening. Moreover, as we only focus on the therapeutic part of the management, we eliminated other sections, *i.e.* list of authors, evaluation, diagnosis and references. The three CPGs have then been compiled into a single document for the further steps of the analysis.
2. *Automatic term extraction.* The compiled document has been submitted to TermoStat which returned a list of candidate terms, sorted by their score of specificity, and associated to their syntactic contexts, *i.e.* expressions surrounding each candidate term.
3. *Manual removal of non-relevant terms.* Meaningless terms such as prepositions, e.g. "of", or units, e.g. "mmHg", have been removed. The remaining candidate terms have been evaluated using syntactic contexts. When a candidate term was considered out of the scope (e.g. "pluridisciplinary approach", "reversible case", "epidemiology"), it was also removed. The whole process led to a subset of terms that were actually related to the therapeutic management of hypertension.
4. *Candidate terms clustering and concepts identification.* This step consists in gathering candidate terms related to a same concept in a bottom-up approach. Once again, syntactic contexts built by TermoStat have been used. For instance, the term "occlusion" is used in only one syntactic context related to "ischemic stroke". Three persons with different backgrounds have independently performed this step (AG, JB, and BS). Resulting clusters have been compared and conflicts if any have been resolved. We finally obtained clusters of terms related to a same concept. For instance, the cluster R7 associated to the concept of "ischemic stroke" is made of the terms "ischemic attack, transient ischemic attack, intracerebral artery occlusion, carotid artery, extracranial carotid, ischemia, ischemic, occlusion".

5. *Building of conceptual coverage.* For each CPGs, identified relevant candidate terms have been mapped to medical concepts, the set of which is called the conceptual coverage of the CPG. The conceptual coverage of the three CPGs have been compared according to set operations.

2. Results

The compilation of the three narrative CPGs is a document containing 11,313 word occurrences. TermoStat identified 723 candidate terms among which 246 were found to be non-relevant and were removed. Then, the 477 remaining terms have been manually grouped into 88 clusters, each cluster being related to a single medical concept. When identifying the conceptual coverage of each CPGs, we found that VR-HTA included 81 concepts, SFHTA included 53 concepts, and CHEP included 73 concepts. Figure 1 quantitatively illustrates the conceptual coverage of each CPGs. It also shows the set of concepts specific to each CPGs.

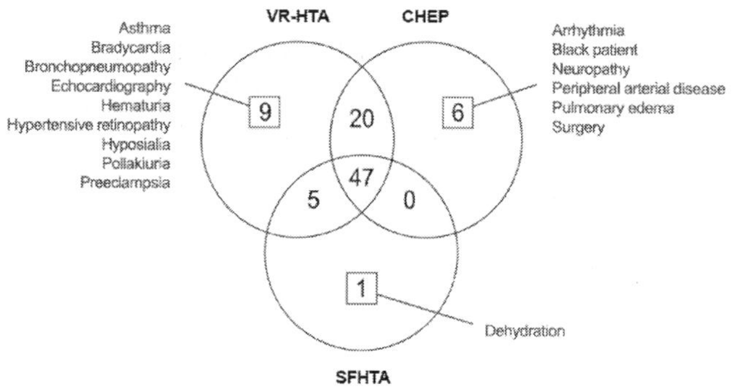

Figure 1. – Distribution of concepts between the three CPGs.

47 concepts (53% of the total) are common to the 3 CPGs; they represent the core concepts of hypertension management. Sixteen concepts (18% of the total) appear in only one guideline: 9 in VR-HTA (56%), 1 in SFHTA (6%), and 6 in CHEP (38%). It should be noticed that the intersection of VR-HTA and CHEP contains 67 concepts and that 98% of the concepts covered by SFHTA are also covered by the union of VR-HTA and CHEP.

3. Discussion

We implemented a semi-automated method using term extraction to characterize the conceptual coverage of the therapeutic part of three CPGs published in French on the management of hypertension in 2013. Only 53% of all the identified concepts are shared by the three CPGs, highlighting common parts but also identifying specificities. Specificities may be explained by multiple factors, such as the authoring country, or the level of generality of texts. For instance, the shortest guideline SFHTA is nearly totally included in VR-HTA and has only one specific medical concept "dehydration". VR-HTA and CHEP, which are both larger documents, share 76% of all medical concepts

(67/88). Their specificities correspond, for VR-HTA, to a focus on specific drug contraindications (asthma, bradycardia, bronchopneumopathy), specific drug side-effects (dry mouth, urinary frequency), an extended set of particular conditions (pre-eclampsia in case of pregnancy), or specific complementary exams (echocardiography, hematuria, retinopathy), and, for CHEP, to additional particular cases (arrhythmia, black patient, neuropathy, peripheral arterial disease, pulmonary edema, surgery).

This work has some limitations. The first one comes from the use of TermoStat. The statistical approach of TermoStat calculates a score for each term from its relative frequency within the processed text with respect to the reference corpus. A term will be highlighted depending on its frequency of occurrence in the text from which it is extracted. We started to process the three CPGs separately and found many false negatives (e.g. creatinemia was found specific of VR-HTA, although existing in the two other CPGs). To counter this problem, we have compiled the three recommendations into a single document for term extraction by TermoStat. The three CPGs have thus been processed in a coherent manner, and biases, if any, are the same for the three documents. Another limitation comes from the subjectivity of manual concepts elicitation although it has been independently done by three persons.

This work is the first step of the analysis of CPGs content. Extending this work by taking into account CPGs written in other languages would require to perform a separate, language-dependent, term extraction, then to map terms to the language-independent concepts. However, the comparison based on the concepts existing in CPGs is not the comparison of the content. Thus, even if concepts are shared, recommendations may be different. We have started to model CPGs knowledge as decision rules, to evaluate to which extent CPGs deliver similar recommendations for similar patients. In this perspective we consider that guideline-specific concepts are an asset that should be used to complete the set of clinical profiles described in CPGs, and enriching the knowledge base of CDSSs thus broadening the coverage of such systems.

References

[1] M.W. Jaspers, M. Smeulers, H. Vermeulen, L.W. Peute, Effects of clinical decision-support systems on practitioner performance and patient outcomes: a synthesis of high-quality systematic review findings, *J Am Med Inform Assoc.*, **18**(3) (2011), 327–34.

[2] B. Séroussi, J. Bouaud, G. Chatellier, Guideline-based modeling of therapeutic strategies in the special case of chronic diseases, *Int J Med Inform* **74**(2-4) (2005), 89–99.

[3] Vidal. Vidal Recos HTA. 2013. [Commercial content available at http://www.vidal.fr/recommandations/1640/hta_hypertension_arterielle/. Last accessed January 6, 2014].

[4] SFHTA. Recommandation sur « La prise en charge de l'hypertension artérielle de l'adulte». 2013. [Available at http://www.sfhta.eu/wp-content/uploads/2012/12/Recommandation-SFHTA-2013-Prise-en-charge-HTA-de-lAdulte.pdf. Last accessed January 6, 2014].

[5] Hypertension Canada. Recommandations 2013 du Programme Éducatif Canadien sur l'Hypertension. 2013. [Available at http://www.hypertension.ca/images/CHEP_2013/2013_CHEPRecsFullVersion_FR_HCP1000.pdf. Last accessed January 6, 2014].

[6] G. Georg, I. Colombet, P. Durieux, J. Ménard, P. Meneton, A comparative analysis of four CPGs for hypertension management, *J Hum Hypertens*, **22**(12) (2008), 829-37

[7] A. Hatsek, O. Young, E. Shalom, Y. Shahar, DeGeL: a clinical-guidelines library and automated guideline-support tools, *Stud Health Technol Inform.* **139** (2008), 203-12.

[8] K. Kaiser, C. Akkaya, S. Miksch, How can information extraction ease formalizing treatment processes in clinical practice guidelines? A method and its evaluation, *Artif Intell Med.* **39**(2) (2007), 151-63, Epub 2006 Sep 8.

[9] P. Drouin, Term extraction using non-technical corpora as a point of leverage. Terminology **9**(1) (2003), 99-115.

Sources of Data, Including Big Data, for Monitoring and Measuring Health and Disease

Cross-Border Challenges in Informatics with a Focus on Disease Surveillance and Utilising Big Data 29
L. Stoicu-Tivadar et al. (Eds.)

doi:10.3233/978-1-61499-389-6-29

Practical Implementation of a Bridge between Legacy EHR System and a Clinical Research Environment

Dina VISHNYAKOVA[a,1], Sylviane BOTTONE[b], Emilie PASCHE[a] and Christian LOVIS[a]
[a] *Division of Medical Information Sciences, University Hospitals and University of Geneva, Switzerland*
[b] *Division of Medical Information Sciences, University Hospitals of Geneva, Switzerland*

Abstract. Employing the bridge between Clinical Information System (CIS) and Clinical Research Environment (CRE) can provide functionality, which is not easily, implemented by traditional legacy EHR system. In this paper, the experience of such implementation at the University Hospitals of Geneva is described. General overview of the mapping of extracted from CIS data to the i2b2 Clinical Data Warehouse is provided. The defined implementation manages to provide the interoperability for the CRE.

Keywords. Data Integration, Clinical Information System, Electronic Health Records, Big Data, Clinical Data Warehouse.

Introduction

The global data double their volume every two years. Furthermore, the increasing of the healthcare data digitization means that healthcare organizations, often, add terabytes of patient records to data centres annually. At present, most of this unstructured data is not used, partly, due to the legacy systems (LS) and mainly they are in sight of regulatory purposes.

A better understanding of data such as to know more about an individual patient or large groups of them and how to use this information provides better, more efficient and cheaper healthcare. Additionally, arose the challenge to reuse clinical information for real-time care or clinical research [1-3]. Furthermore, the process of health information exchange, necessary for getting the patient data is neither easy nor simple. For example, one electronic health record (EHR) system uses "hypertension" and another one may call it "elevated blood pressure". To solve this problem, the standards such as ICD-9/10, SNOMED CT, LOINC and many more are used [4]. The advantage of the standardization is to facilitate the research query process.

The analysis of big data is of high priority but the processing of such data is a major challenge. Here, one of the major problems is a data lookup in a legacy EHR system. Physicians and research stuff need that patient information is accessible

---

[1] Corresponding Author.

regardless its way of keeping records in current EHR system. Mostly, the data are left within the legacy system, requiring users to login to another system in order to access all relevant patient information. This process is very expensive and time-consuming.

Here, we present the bridge methodology, between legacy EHR and a CRE used at the University Hospitals of Geneva (Hôpitaux Universitaires de Genève, HUG) that closely conjoins with the hospital clinical information systems.

1. Data and Methods

The association of 8 hospitals of Geneva and 40 ambulatories spread throughout the territory of the canton merged into the first university hospital in Switzerland, the HUG.

HUG is comprised of more than 2,000 beds. According to annual statistics, approximately 60,000 admissions and over 900,000 outpatient visits took place. There were over 6,000,000 laboratory testing done in 2013. The total number of full-time employees is about 9,000, where the number of physicians is about 1.300.

1.1. Design objectives

The design of the bridge methodology between legacy EHR and a CRE was focused around several goals. The primary goal is to provide a secure and clear representation of patient information for research purposes. Moreover, in healthcare domain, the cross-border integration of data is a challenge. Due to the ethical reasons, data providers are not allowed to store patient data outside of their hospital infrastructure (Intranet).

Furthermore, due to a high-level protection to preserve system stability the real time analysis/visualisation of data cannot be applied. Such data representation needed to be based on a software framework that is secure and could be easily extended.

1.2. Implementation tools

Respecting all constrains, described above, it was decided to use Open Source software and the i2b2 (Informatics for Integrating Biology & the Bedside) framework. The design of i2b2 is based on web services that provide securable remote access to its various parts [5]. Moreover, researchers can use i2b2 to perform research queries of de-identified data.

Clinical Information System (CIS) of HUG include different database management systems and access protocols. In order to provide a homogenous access to the information, the i2b2 server placed between CIS and the i2b2 client or a so-called query endpoint, see Fig. 1. The endpoint is responsible for the resulting information representation extracted from the i2b2 server. The i2b2 server is periodically fulfilled by pre-constructed ETL processes in the following order: 1) retrieve the content of CIS 2) perform model transformation 3) load data into the i2b2 CDW.

The first principle step at ETL stage is to pseudonymise sensitive patients' data [8] such as patient ID number, Episodes of care, date of birth. Despite the ability of i2b2 to restrict/grant access to identified data within its security policies, a pseudonymisation step took place during the extraction phase. In all the circumstances, by doing so, the restitution of patient identifiers is reversible only by means of authorities that are responsible for the data extraction phase. In our case, a hash encryption function is

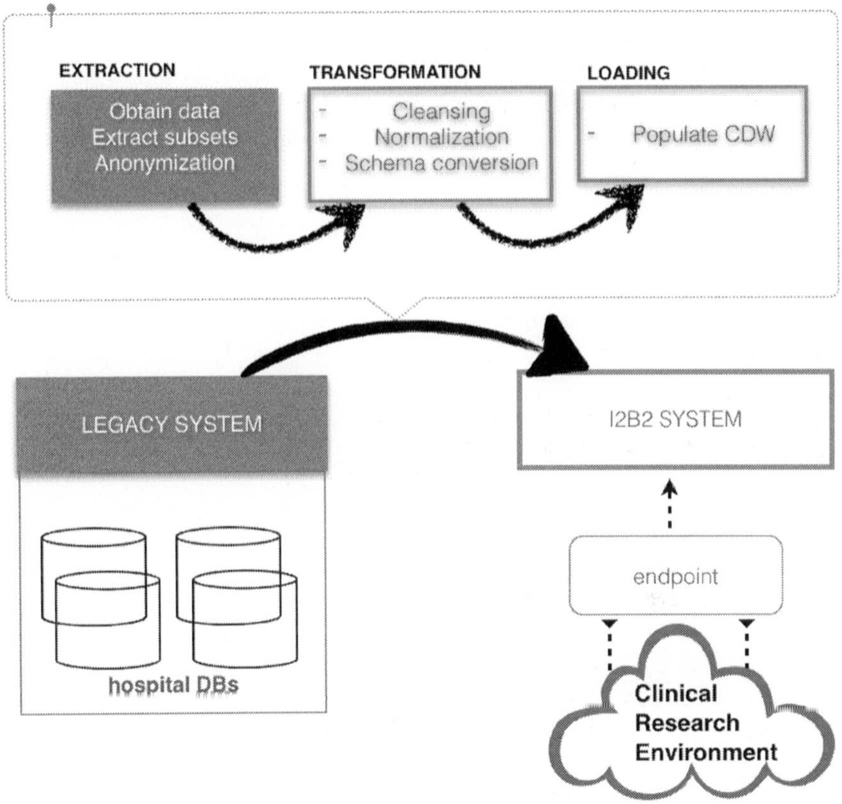

Figure 1. Information Workflow. The Intranet components are shown in colour.

used at the Extraction phase. The mapping table with keys to identified data never leaves the Intranet location of HUG. Such data as international standardization codes are available without constraints.

1.3. Data Mapping

The i2b2 schema is represented as a five-axis star: PATIENT, VISIT, OBSERVATION, CONCEPT and PROVIDER.

The HUG CIS data corresponding to PATIENT, VISIT and PROVIDER can be easily integrated directly to the i2b2 schema while to fulfil CONCEPT and OBSERVATION is a challenging task.

The mapping of CONCEPT dimension, which consists of lab tests, medications and etc., is challenging. HUG data are not all standardized in accordance with the international standardization codes. Moreover, i2b2 keeps a tree structure of concepts in its schema it is necessary to return data records containing the name of concept, the id for the concept and ids of concept's ancestors. Nevertheless, it is not exceptional to find a free form text with the optional standardisation codes.

In order to avoid missing important concepts, it was necessary to add additional values to standard dictionaries. This required a separate concept table that stores new repository codes for data that have no standard dictionary code. In some cases of free text mapping, specific algorithms such as described in [4,6,7] based on biomedical terminologies (SNOMED CT, NEWT and etc.) were implemented to perform term normalization of data retrieved from CIS.

Most data are stored in the OBSERVATION table. In this table every row is an observation on a patient (Diagnosis, Procedures, Laboratory data and etc.). Each row correlates with one observation about a patient made during a visit. There are several requirements to the patient observation such as: to be related to a patient, to contain temporal information (e.g. start and end date), to be related to concepts defined in CONCEPT dimension.

2. Discussion and Conclusion

To date, there is no optimal solution for the legacy system replacement. In many research cases the incompatibility of data in such systems becomes a time-consuming challenge for the research communities. On other hand the simplicity of data representation by such system as i2b2 opens the horizons for the effective clinical data management. By building the bridge between the LS and research environment the achievements in tasks such as clinical investigations/studies, quality management and etc. become feasible. This type of bridging omits the need in global data mapping strategies, costly extraction of relevant clinical data from source systems and etc.

Currently, this way of bridging is involved in the framework of one of the largest European public/private partnership projects in the eHealth area - EHR4CR [2] (Electronic Health Records for Clinical Research). This project aims to provide adaptable, scalable and interoperable solutions for reusing data from EHR systems for the clinical research. The CRE of EHR4CR avoids a global data model representation, which makes possible to integrate different sources of data and to ensure the scalability. The i2b2 CDW settled by HUG is only required to have the corresponding endpoint and the corresponding mapping of added sources to EHR4CR data codes.

By bridging data the quality of information can also be improved as the data from different EHR systems is integrated through a standardized process of data extraction, normalization, transformation, and loading (ETL). The resulting consistency of data may increase research confidence as the bridging can eliminate the conflicting results that are often reported due to the different data sources or different ETL processes.

We will continue to deploy services to update the HUG CDW continuously and to evaluate its usefulness, advantages and disadvantages.

Acknowledgements

The research leading to these results has received support from the Innovative Medicines Initiative Joint Undertaking under grant agreement n° [115489], resources of

[2] The IMI EHR4CR Project runs over 5 years (2011-2015). This project involves 33 partners (academic and industrial). More information at http://www.ehr4cr.eu

which are composed of financial contribution from the European Union's Seventh Framework Programme (FP7/2007-2013) and EFPIA companies' in kind contribution.

References

[1] H.U. Prokosch, T. Ganslandt, Perspectives for medical informatics. Reusing the electronic medical record for clinical research, *Methods Inf Med.* **48**(2009), 38–44.

[2] C.Ohmann, W. Kuchinke, Future developments of medical informatics from the viewpoint of networked clinical research. Interoperaility and Integration, *Methods Inf. Med.* **48 (2009),** 45-54

[3] P. Knaup, O. Bott, C. Kohl, C. Lovis, S. Garde, Electronic patient records: moving from islands and bridges towards electronic health records for continuity of care, Yearb Med Inform, 2007, 34-46.

[4] P. Ruch, J. Gobeill, C. Lovis, A. Geissbühler, Automatic medical encoding with SNOMED categories, *BMC medical informatics and decision making,* **8** (2008), S6.

[5] S.N. Murphy, M. Mendis, K.Hackett, R. Kuttan, W. Pan, L.C. Phillips, H.C. Chueh, Architecture of the open-source clinical research chart from Informatics for Integrating Biology and the Bedside, *In AMIA Annual Symposium Proceedings (2007). American Medical Informatics Association.*, 548

[6] D. Vishnyakova, E. Pasche, C. Lovis, P. Ruch Utilization of ontology look-up services in information retrieval for biomedical literature, *Studies in health technology and informatics* **186** (2012), 155-159.

[7] Y. Vishnyakov, R. Vishnyakov Semantic proximity in information retrieval and documents classification In Computational Intelligence and Informatics, *IEEE 14th International Symposium on* (2013), 131-134.

[8] P. Ruch, R. H. Baud, A. M. Rassinoux, P. Bouillon, G. Robert, Medical document anonymization with a semantic lexicon, *In Proceedings of the AMIA Symposium, American Medical Informatics Association* (2000), 729.

Cross-Border Challenges in Informatics with a Focus on Disease Surveillance and Utilising Big Data
L. Stoicu-Tivadar et al. (Eds.)

doi:10.3233/978-1-61499-389-6-35

Automated Detection of Ambiguity in BI-RADS Assessment Categories in Mammography Reports

Selen BOZKURT [a,1] and Daniel RUBIN [b]
[a] *Akdeniz University, Antalya, Turkey*
[b] *Stanford University, Stanford, CA*

Abstract. An unsolved challenge in biomedical natural language processing (NLP) is detecting ambiguities in the reports that can help physicians to improve report clarity. Our goal was to develop NLP methods to tackle the challenges of identifying ambiguous descriptions of the laterality of BI-RADS Final Assessment Categories in mammography radiology reports. We developed a text processing system that uses a BI-RADS ontology we built as a knowledge source for automatic annotation of the entities in mammography reports relevant to this problem. We used the GATE NLP toolkit and developed customized processing resources for report segmentation, named entity recognition, and detection of mismatches between BI-RADS Final Assessment Categories and mammogram laterality. Our system detected 55 mismatched cases in 190 reports and the accuracy rate was 81%. We conclude that such NLP techniques can detect ambiguities in mammography reports and may reduce discrepancy and variability in reporting.

Keywords. Breast Imaging Reporting and Data System (BI-RADS), Information Extraction, Natural Language Processing, Imaging Informatics, Breast.

Introduction

The interpretation of mammography images is challenged by variability among radiologists, and the development of new methods to improve radiologist performance is needed [1-2]. An initial step to reduce radiologist variation is to standardize the vocabulary used in mammography reports. Therefore, The American College of Radiology (ACR) developed Breast Imaging-Reporting and Data System (BI-RADS). It is called a "system" because it contains several important components, including 1) a lexicon of descriptors, 2) a recommended reporting structure, including "Final Assessment Categories" with accompanying management recommendations, and 3) a framework for data collection and auditing [3]. Final Assessment Categories are summary codes that indicate the radiologist's level of suspicion a malignancy is present: BI-RADS 0 Need Additional Imaging Evaluation and/or Prior Mammograms for Comparison, BI-RADS 1 Negative, BI-RADS 2 Benign, BI-RADS 3 Probably Benign, BI-RADS 4 Suspicious Abnormality, BI-RADS 5 Highly Suggestive of Malignancy, BI-RADS 6 Known Biopsy Proven Malignancy. BI-RADS terms have

[1] Corresponding Author.

also been developed to describe breast density, lesion features, impression, and recommendations, and the system has been revised and updated many times [3-6].

While adoption of BI-RADS can help standardize the vocabulary and reduce the variation in mammography reporting, it is not a decision support system (DSS) for mammography, though others have used it as a key ingredient of DSS [3]. Several substantial efforts have been undertaken in creating DSS for mammography; however, few have been adopted in clinical practice, largely due to the challenge of not disrupting the workflow. DSS usually entail recording the mammography results in a structured reporting system or as a separate workflow, which is time-consuming. A potentially better approach would be to incorporate DSS directly into the workflow by inserting it into the radiology report generation process. Since radiology reports are created as unstructured text reports, in this strategy Natural language processing (NLP) techniques are needed to extract structured information from reports to provide the inputs to DSS. Therefore we are developing NLP methods to use to extract the BI-RADS Final Assessment Categories from free-text mammography reports in order to provide input data to DSS to reduce variability in mammography interpretations.

A particular challenge to using NLP for DSS is that separate BI-RADS Final Assessment Categories may not be reported for the left and right breast separately. In such cases, the laterality of the Final Assessment Category (i.e., which breast was reported to have a given category) is ambiguous. This can cause clinical confusion as well as hamper ability to use these reports in decision support systems.

Our goals was to develop NLP methods to tackle the challenges of ambiguous descriptions of the laterality of BI-RADS Final Assessment Categories in mammography, as well as to extract them, to enable a future system to alert the radiologist if there is any ambiguity in reporting BI-RADS Final Assessment Categories.

1. Method

The BI-RADS terminology is a simple list and it has no information about radiology report structure. We constructed a “BI-RADS ontology” which contains mammography Imaging Observations (Conditions, problems, and etc.), Location (laterality, clock face location and etc.) and Report entities.

Using the BI-RADS ontology, we created a text processing pipeline (Figure 1) which uses the ontology as a knowledge source for automatic annotation of the entities in mammography reports, as described below. Our pipeline performs the following tasks (Figure 1): (1) tokenization of words, numbers and punctuation; (2) part of speech tagging, (3) stemming; (4) matching tokens in the text to entities in the BI-RADS ontology; (5) report section recognition and segmentation, annotation of each sentence in each section and also detection of report title, (6) named entity recognition of BI-RADS Final Assessment Categories. The title of a radiology report usually describes whether the left breast, right breast, or both breasts were imaged, while the Impression section describes the BI-RADS Final Assessment Categories and laterality (the category for each breast). Thus, the named entity recognition step is applied to the Impression section and both named entity recognition of laterality detection are applied to both the impression section and the report title.

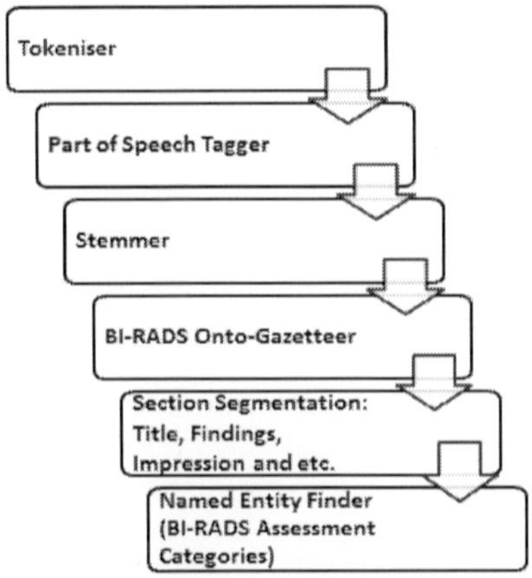

Figure 1. The Pipeline.

We built our system using the GATE (General Architecture for Text Engineering) NLP toolkit [4]. GATE is an open source framework and also provides several configurable processing resources which we assembled into a processing pipeline to parse words, numbers, and punctuation (Tokenizer) and annotate documents based on keyword lists (Gazetteer lists). In addition, GATE provides regular expression pattern matching engine called Java Annotation Patterns Engine (JAPE), which is a multi-pass regular expression parser tightly integrated with GATE's document annotation representation.

In addition to use GATE's built in processing resources such as Tokenizer and stemmer, we implemented a series of custom regular expression-based rules using JAPE grammar, which matches tokens in the text to entities in the BI-RADS ontology using the Onto-Gazetteer. This module thus accomplishes ontological linkage of entities in the text to the ontology. For the section segmentation and named entity finder, we developed custom components by creating JAPE grammars.

- **Section Segmentation.** Although radiology reports are free text, they are loosely structured in terms of sections, and each section has its own heading in most cases that can be used to unambiguously identify it. We developed a processing resource in GATE that recognizes section headings and uses them to segment the reports into sections.
- **Recognizing Named Entities.** This was developed to capture BI-RADS Final Assessment Categories and the laterality information in impression sentences or report title then tag them as Assessment or Laterality named entities. The module uses the BI-RADS Onto-Gazetteer to tag all BI-RADS descriptors in the text.
- **Identification of Laterality.** We created rules to associate BI-RADS Assessment Categories and the report title with laterality entity.
- **Data.** We developed our system based on analysis of 35 example reports (5 reports for each BI-RADS Final Assessment Category). These reports were not used in the evaluation of our system. To test our system, we created a corpus containing 190 radiology reports of mammography having a balanced representation of the different BI-RADS classification codes. In all reports in our database, each section had its own heading and the report title was the first sentence of the report.

- **Evaluation.** We compared the impression section, report title and BI-RADS Final Assessment Categories detected by our system with the gold standard. We also compared the laterality reported in the title of the report with the BI-RADS Final Assessment Category reported in the report impression section. If they did not match, we reported those cases as ambiguous.

2. Results

Our preliminary report set contained 190 reports. The report title, impression section, named entities related to BI-RADS Final Assessment Categories, and laterality were detected perfectly in each report. In addition, laterality related the title was detected correctly for each report. Our system could not find any laterality information for BI-RADS Final Assessment Category in only two reports.

Out of all reports, 54 (28%) of reports were bilateral mammography reports and 136 (71%) of them were unilateral mammography reports. Eight reports did not have a title; therefore, they did not have laterality specified for the entire report.

In 87 reports, laterality of BI-RADS Final Assessment Categories were not defined, and in 45 reports laterality in title were not declared. In terms of ambiguity, in 55 reports laterality information in title and BI-RADS Final Assessment Category did not match; thus our system correctly identified 45 of these cases of report ambiguity. Six of 54 bilateral mammography reports only included BI-RADS Final Assessment Category for one of the breasts. In one report, although it was a left mammography report, BI-RADS Final Assessment Category was given for right breast, so our system detected this ambiguity correctly. Overall, the accuracy of our system in detecting ambiguity in laterality of BI-RADS Final Assessment Categories was 81%.

3. Discussion

To allow concise and unambiguous understanding reports and to reduce variability in reporting, standardized BI-RADS Final Assessment Category codes (0 to 6) are used in routine radiology practice [5]. Although it is critical that the Final Assessment Category result in the correct action, recent studies showed that there is still intra- and inter-observer variability in mammography interpretations based on BI-RADS classification codes, and new researches are necessary to solve those problems [6].

Table 1. Laterality in title and laterality of BI-RADS final assessment classification crosstab.

	Laterality for BI-RADS Final Assessment Categories				
Laterality in Title	Not Identified	Left	Right	Both	Total
Not Identified	41	-	3*	1*	45
Unilateral	4*	6	1	-	11
Left	2	41	1*	-	45
Right	5*		23		28
Bilateral	35*	1*	5*	13	54
Total	87	48	33	14	182

* Ambiguous cases

In terms of ambiguities in mammography reporting, we only focused on detecting mismatches between the laterality of BI-RADS Final Assessment Categories. This is clearly only a small subset of all such ambiguities, but we believe our methods are extensible and can be expanded to detecting other ambiguities that may be specified in the future. To identify ambiguities in BI-RADS Final Assessment Codes and laterality in mammography reports, we developed an NLP system based on a rule-based approach. Since our system only recognizes one type of ambiguity, it will be necessary to add additional rules in the future to detect other possible ambiguities.

Despite the apparent high accuracy of our system, our methods have several limitations. First, in all reports in our database, each section had its own heading and the report title was the first sentence of the report. Therefore, our method might not work well in other types of reports in which section headers are absent. In addition, although the regular expressions we used seemed to work well for detecting laterality and BI-RADS Final Assessment Codes, our approach is highly domain-specific and might not be generalizable to other applications without substantial revisions to our processing modules. On the other hand, since our system was developed in the modular platform of GATE, and we have encapsulated the domain-specific processing JAPE processing resources whose regular expressions are compact and human-readable, we believe such extensions are practical in the future.

4. Conclusion

We have developed a system to detect potential ambiguities in the laterality of BI-RADS Final Assessment Categories. Our system detected 55 ambiguities in 190 reports, with an overall accuracy of 81%. Such NLP techniques to detect ambiguities in clinical reports may reduce discrepancy and variability in reporting. We are planning to extend this study to find and extract additional types of entities as well as to extract relationships among entities as well as the location of abnormalities reported in mammography, to provide the inputs to a decision support system that is linked to reporting. Ambiguity detection will be an important feature of such a system to provide feedback to radiologists. We will also be conducting a more complete evaluation in a larger corpus of reports.

References

[1] G.E. Joann, K.W. Carolyn, H.L. Carol, H.H. Debra, R.F. Alvan, Variability in radiologists' interpretations of mammograms, *N Engl J Med.* **331**(22)(1994), 1493-1499.

[2] K. Kerlikowske, D. Grady, J. Barclay et al., Variability and accuracy in mammographic interpretation using the American College of Radiology Breast Imaging Reporting and Data System, *J Natl Cancer Inst* **90**(23)(1998), 1801-1809.

[3] E.S. Burnside, E.A. Sickles, L.W. Bassett et al., The ACR BI-RADS experience: learning from history, *J Am Coll Radiol* **6**(12)(2009), 851-860.

[4] L. Liberman, J.H. Menell, Breast imaging reporting and data system (BI-RADS), *Radiol Clin North Am* **40**(3)(2002), 409-455.

[5] H. Cunningham, GATE, A General Architecture for Text Engineering, *Computers and the Humanities* **36**(2) (2002), 223-254.

[6] American College of Radiology, Breast Imaging Reporting and Data System Atlas (BI-RADS Atlas), 2003.

L. Stoicu-Tivadar et al. (Eds.)

doi:10.3233/978-1-61499-389-6-41

Data and Knowledge in Medical Distributed Applications

Alexandru SERBAN[a,1], Mihaela CRIŞAN-VIDA[a] and Lăcrămioara STOICU-TIVADAR[a]
[a] *Department of Automation and Applied Informatics, University Politehnica Timişoara, Romania*

Abstract. Building a clinical decision support system (CDSS) capable to collect process and diagnose data from the patients automatically, based on information, symptoms and investigations is one of the current challenges for researchers and medical science. The purpose of the current study is to design a cloud-based CDSS to improve patient safety, quality of care and organizational efficiency. It presents the design of a cloud-based application system using a medical based approach, which covers different diseases to diagnosis, differentiated on most important pathologies. Using online questionnaires, traditional and new data will be collected from patients. After data input, the application will formulate a presumptive diagnosis and will direct patients to the correspondent department. A questionnaire will dynamically ask questions about the interface, and functionality improvements. Based on the answers, the functionality of the system and the user interface will be improved considering the real needs expressed by the end-users. The cloud-based CDSS, as a useful tool for patients, physicians and healthcare providers involves the computer support in the diagnosis of different pathologies and an accurate automatic differential diagnostic system.

Keywords. Cloud-based application, patients, physicians, healthcare providers, clinical decision support systems, interfaces

Introduction

Clinical decision support systems (CDSS) are important tools to improve health care outcomes and reduce preventable medical adverse events [1]. Based on literature, a CDSS can provide software-based, healthcare-related advice to assist doctors and nurses in making decisions and developing solutions, and is often used in complex or non-routine situations [2]. Decision support in the cloud is feasible and may be a reasonable path toward achieving better support of clinical decision-making across the widest range of health care providers [3]. CDS entails providing clinicians, patients, and other healthcare stakeholders with pertinent knowledge and person-specific information, intelligently filtered or presented at appropriate times, to enhance health and healthcare [4]. CDS has been shown to improve prescribing practices, reduce serious medication errors, enhance delivery of preventive care services, and improve guidelines adherence, and likely results in lasting improvements in clinical practice [5].

---

[1]Corresponding Author.

Currently, electronic knowledge bases, together with inference procedures offer many possibilities for the support of medical decision-making, mainly in regard to interactive diagnostic work-up, but also the selection of the most suitable treatment plan, and are known also as Computer-Based Medical Decision Support Systems (CBMDSS) [6].

Until now, different cloud decision support applications were described: the Clinfowiki, a world-accessible wiki for developing decision support content; Partners Healthcare eRooms, web-based tools for developing decision support within a single organization; and Epic Systems Corporation's Community Library, a repository for sharing decision support content for customers of a single clinical system vendor [7].

A meta-regression of 162 randomised trials identified factors that differentiate between effective and ineffective computerised CDSS in terms of improvements in the process of care or in patient outcomes. The authors observed that presenting decision support within electronic charting or order entry systems are associated with failure compared with other ways of delivering advice. Odds of success were greater for systems that required practitioners to provide reasons when over-riding advice than for systems that did not [8]. A recently systematic review that included 148 randomized, controlled trials evaluated the effect of CDSSs on clinical outcomes, health care processes, workload and efficiency, patient satisfaction, cost, and provider use and implementation. The authors concluded that both commercially and locally developed CDSSs are effective at improving health care process measures across diverse settings, but evidence for clinical, economic, workload and efficiency outcomes remains sparse [9].

The purpose of the current study is to present a new cloud-based CDSS designed to improve patient safety, quality of care and organizational efficiency.

1. Methods

This paper presents the design of a new cloud-based CDSS centered on patients, physicians and healthcare providers (Figure 1.).

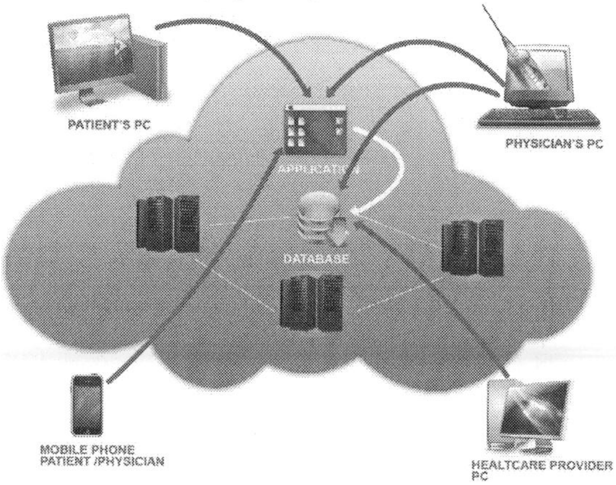

Figure 1. The concept of the application

Firstly, the application will collect data from patients like age, gender, race, ethnicity, socio-economic status, anthropometric parameters, leisure-time physical activity, cigarettes smoking, and alcohol and caffeine consumption behavior through specific questions through a website. Secondly, the cloud-based CDSS will allow physicians to insert more data like laboratory analysis and different investigations if these exist, for a more accurate diagnosis (Figure 2.).

Physicians may input information in the system and the decision support system software will output an appropriate diagnosis, for them to act on it that they find are relevant.

The patients will have the possibility to access the application via an Internet browser, from any device connected to Internet.

The application will provide the connection among family physicians, specialty physicians, hospitals and patients to achieve improved clinical outcomes while reducing costs.

Communication between different components is using HL7 Clinical Document Architecture (HL7 CDA), a document markup standard that specifies the structure and semantics of "clinical documents" for the purpose of exchange between healthcare providers and patients [11]. It includes text, images, multimedia content or sounds. The information is sent using XML in CDA format.

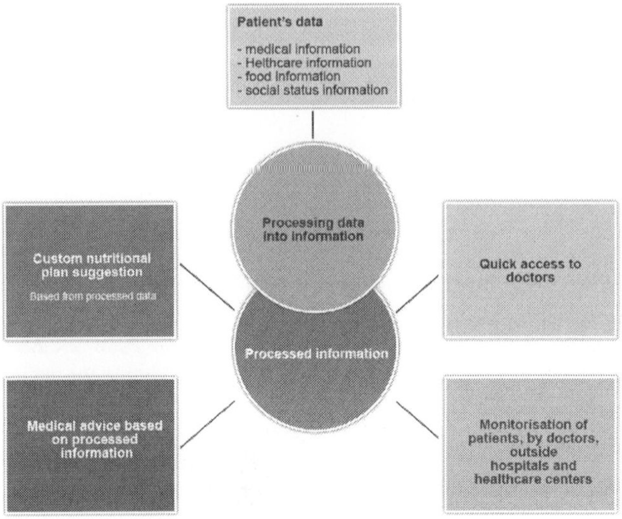

Figure 2. The stucture of the cloud-based CDSS

As innovation for *user-experience design*, the cloud-based CDSS will create an attractive design concept using an attractive appearance, it will use graphic symbols to guide the user within the application it will use multimedia elements (audio, video, and photo) for easy use and quick application and a range of fonts as legible.

As innovation for *information architecture*, a navigation structure of the application as intuitive as possible will be created. The user will be able to quickly access desired information without accessing intermediate pages. A “sitemap" that allow users to quickly access desired information will be implemented. A smart display of errors will be designed to help the user in resolving different issues. Error messages should be short and concise and will provide solutions to problems encountered. The navigation system will be interactive, allowing quickly access to desired information.

Search engine application information will help users to easy find and access information.

As innovation on application development, the cloud-based CDSS will be accessed quickly and easily, both on PCs and on mobile phones based as patient-centered application system. The application will be created on a modular system that will allow further development without much technical interventions. The data will be stored in a secure database, on a functional server 24/7, 365/365. The services will be modeled associated with the application. An automatic analysis and interpretation of data recorded in the system will be implemented. The system developed will allow exporting processed data in different file formats. Using Generic Component Model will be created a model of interconnection of cloud-base applications: applications for easy diagnosis and for nutritional plan.

The development of cloud-based CDSS will be easily adapted and personalized for healthcare providers needs, providing an interactive service patient-centered home type who can diagnose, monitor and assist patients enrolled in the system development even outside hospitals. The databases will use new concepts like *big time* to address to the patients.

A questionnaire will dynamically ask questions about the user interface, and functionality improvements. Physicians will report if the design process is user-friendly, accurate and easy to use. Based on the answers, the functionality of the system and the interface will be further improved considering the real needs expressed by the end-users.

2. Discussion

A cloud-based CDSS delivered using information systems, with the electronic medical record as the platform, will provide decision makers with tools making in order to achieve large gains in performance, narrow gaps between knowledge and practice, and improve safety [10]. The number of cloud decision support applications is highly increasing. Our application is an example of cloud-based CDSS that analyzes patient data stored in electronic medical records and administrative data systems and formulates a presumptive diagnosis and a life-style changing plan.

The application will be designed from three different points of view: advantages for physicians, for patients and for healthcare providers.

From the technological view, the cloud-based CDSS developed for healthcare providers and doctors will allow medical data storage, easy access of users (patients) trough a web interface and easy access from PC, Laptop and Smart Phones.

From the medical view, the cloud-based CDSS will help physicians to easy access patient's folders and diagnostic history and to monitor the patients, even outside of healthcare centers, providing a 7-days-a-week collection of real-time data. The application will assist physicians and nurses at point of care by using patient data for determination of appropriate diagnoses for the patients, in crucial decision management and predictive analytics, to enhance health outcomes. The cloud-based CDSS will eliminate typing errors, usually seen in manual collection data and will allow online communication between patients and doctors. The cloud-based CDSS will spare time for patients, considering actually barriers to attend a doctor: lack of knowledge about diseases, transportation, inconvenient times, busy schedules, space limitations, long waiting lists and intensive time commitments. Our application will help patients to access medical services more easily. Patients could receive an advised medical help quickly, also a nutritional plan suggestion based on input data considering highly personalized, evidence-based care patient characteristics. The patients could be monitored even outside of healthcare providers. The cloud-based CDSS will automatically schedule the patients for regulate controls, month by month, by sending them online reminders. The advantage for healthcare providers will be the possibility of customizing of the application considering the needs.

Conclusions

A web-based decision support in the cloud can help physicians and healthcare providers to improve the quality of medical services by increasing the efficiency of operations and sharing information across geographic locations while reducing costs and also patients in accessing medical services more easily. The application is under development.

References

[1] M.J. Yuan, G.M. Finley, J. Long, C. Mills, R.K. Johnson, Evaluation of user interface and workflow design of a bedside nursing clinical decision support system, I*nteractive journal of medical research,* (2013), 2:e4.

[2] A.E. de Vries, M.H. van der Wal, M.M. Nieuwenhuis, R.M. de Jong, R.B. van Dijk, T. Jaarsma et al., Perceived barriers of heart failure nurses and cardiologists in using clinical decision support systems in the treatment of heart failure patients, *BMC medical informatics and decision making* **13** (2013), 54.

[3] B.E. Dixon, L. Simonaitis, H.S. Goldberg, M.D. Paterno, M. Schaeffer, T. Hongsermeier et al,. A pilot study of distributed knowledge management and clinical decision support in the cloud, *Artificial intelligence in medicine* (2013).

[4] J.A. Osheroff, J.M. Teich, B. Middleton, E.B. Steen, A. Wright, D.E. Detmer, A roadmap for national action on clinical decision support, *Journal of the American Medical Informatics Association : JAMIA* **14** (2007), 141-145.

[5] K.M. Augestad, G. Berntsen, K. Lassen, J.G. Bellika, R. Wootton, R.O. Lindsetmo, Standards for reporting randomized controlled trials in medical informatics: a systematic review of CONSORT adherence in RCTs on clinical decision support, *Journal of the American Medical Informatics Association : JAMIA* **19** (2012), 13-21.

[6] W. Tomaszewski, Computer-Based Medical Decision Support System based on guidelines, clinical pathways and decision nodes, *Acta of bioengineering and biomechanics / Wroclaw University of Technology* **14** (2012), 107-16.

[7] A. Wright, D.W. Bates, B. Middleton, T. Hongsermeier, V. Kashyap, S.M. Thomas et al., Creating and sharing clinical decision support content with Web 2.0: Issues and examples, *Journal of biomedical informatics* **42** (2009), 334-46.

[8] P.S. Roshanov, N. Fernandes, J.M. Wilczynski, B.J. Hemens, J.J. You, S.M. Handler et al., Features of effective computerised clinical decision support systems: meta-regression of 162 randomised trials, *BMJ,* **346** (2013), f657.

[9] T.J. Bright, A.Wong, R. Dhurjati, E. Bristow, L. Bastian, R.R. Coeytaux et al., Effect of clinical decision-support systems: a systematic review, *Annals of internal medicine* **157** (2012), 29-43.

[10] D.W. Bates, G.J. Kuperman, S. Wang, T. Gandhi, A. Kittler, L. Volk et al., Ten commandments for effective clinical decision support: making the practice of evidence-based medicine a reality, *Journal of the American Medical Informatics Association : JAMIA* **10** (2003), 523-30.

[11] HL7 Clinical Document Arhitecture, http://www.hl7.org (accessed December 2013).

Cross-Border Challenges in Informatics with a Focus on Disease Surveillance and Utilising Big Data
L. Stoicu-Tivadar et al. (Eds.)

doi:10.3233/978-1-61499-389-6-47

Computer Assisted Treatment Prediction of Low Back Pain Pathologies

Norbert GAL[a,1], Vasile STOICU-TIVADAR[a], Diana ANDREI[b], Dan Ion NEMEŞ[b] and Emanuela NĂDĂŞAN[b]

[a] *"Politehnica" University of Timişoara, Department of Automation and Applied Informatics, Faculty of Automation and Computers*

[b] *City Emergency Hospital – Medical Rehabilitation and Rheumatology Department Victor Babeş University of Medicine and Pharmacy Timişoara, Romania*

Abstract. The paper presents a fuzzy inference system based prediction with the role to determine the appropriate action for patients that presents lower back pain. If not treated correctly lower back pain can degenerate in various diseases. The system infers three possible actions: (1) spinal cord surgery, (2) medication combined with exercises and (3) no action needed. The system takes in consideration the age and sex of the patient, a pain intensity parameter, the metabolic rate of the patient and mobility parameters from the Zebris Mobility device. In total 243 rules have been formulated but only 21% of the rules suggests surgery. The initial results are promising; there is a correlation of 0.83% between the control results and the results from the system.

Keywords. Lower back pain, Medication, Surgery, Fuzzy systems, Quality of life.

Introduction

Intervertebral disc degeneration is characterized by dehydration of the pulposus nucleus and annulus fibrosus wear as a result of multiple mechanical and biochemical factors. A number of degenerative changes can be described as processes of destabilization followed by re-stabilizing processes.

This leads to a "prominent" or "encapsulated hernia" of the annulus fibrosus towards the vertebral hole or root canal. If the means of the ring contention lose their stability, the nuclear material can herniate. This is the so-called "real hernia" or "non encapsulated hernia"[1, 2].

It has been shown that annulus fibrosus presents at its exterior free nerve endings and vascular channels, thus affecting these tissues, with or without migration of nuclear material was proposed as a major cause for low back pain (LBP). The concept of the disk prominence, which results from the internal disjunction of the intervertebral disk, was

[1] Corresponding Author.

investigated as a primary major cause for low back pain [3]. The disc space obstruction associated to degenerative intervertebral disc changes influences the mechanical joint movement and postulated, as a major cause of segmental instability, can also be associated to low back pain.

The diagnosis is difficult because of the multitude of anatomical elements that overlap in the lower back. In most cases, back pain is not the result of a single injury but an accumulation of mechanical stress and incorrect postures sites over several hours, days, weeks or even years. These activities include:

- Prolonged static postures such as "the state in a wound"
- Bending forward
- Repetitive lifting weights
- Incorrect posture and incorrect body mechanics during household and professional activities

After diagnosis establishment, a medical treatment (usually AINS - Non-inflammatory drugs), rest and activity restriction is recommended to the patient. If satisfactory results are not obtained in a week, the patient is sent to a recovery service. Essentially an early diagnosis, a compliant patient and a competent physician can substantially influence the result of disease ("disease outcome") and its quality of life [4, 5, 6, 7]. The treatment remains at the boundary between internal medicine and surgery and requires knowledge of pathogenesis and the natural development of osteonecrosis.

Why do we want a soft prediction? The answer is to have an accurate diagnostic for a quicker and safer treatment. The patient will be measured using Zebris (mobility and posture) [8], will respond to the questionnaire and the daily activity will be computed. With the help of our software, the patient will return very quickly to a normal, fulfilling and independent life.

1. Measured data types

Four types of data will be investigated for each patient: demographic data to identify the gender and age of the patient, the status of the disability (3 degrees), and the daily activity expressed in calories (24 possibilities) and the mobility degree measured using the Zebris device (minimum/ maximum – 3 values).

1.1. Range of motion

The Zebris Mobility (ZM) facility measures the minimum and maximum values reflecting the mobility of the spinal cord when the patient performs flexion, extension and rotation.

The results of these measurements are six arrays that will reflect the degree of mobility associated with the patient. At 20ms intervals the deviation of the body from the normal stationary position recorded. A patient executes various numbers of repetitions of the same exercise. In this case the interested measurement is the mean value of the maximums and minimums of each repetition.

The mathematical formula to calculate the mean minimum and maximum values are the following:

$$F_{max} = \frac{\sum_{i=1}^{n} rep\_max_i}{n} \quad (1),$$

$$F_{min} = \frac{\sum_{i=1}^{n} rep\_min_i}{n} \quad (2),$$

where F_{max} and F_{min} are the interested measures for the flexion exercises, n is the number of repetitions, *rep_max* and *rep_min* are the maximum and minimum values in the repetition.

In the same way the minimum and maximum values are calculated for the rotation and laterality features. The obtained values are for each exercise is divided in 3 parts:

- Flexion: <80° pathologic, 80°-90° normal, >90° pathologic
- Extension: <20° pathologic, 20°-30° normal, >30° pathologic
- Rotation: <30° pathologic, 30°-45° normal, >45° pathologic.

1.2. Pain intensity parameter

The pain intensity parameter is calculated using a set of 10 questions presented below. Our questionnaire is adapted after the Oswestry scale and Quebec scale [9, 10]. These questions investigate the ability of a person to perform daily basic tasks. Each answer is scored from 0 to 5 considering the difficulty of carrying out each task, where 5 is the worst case scenario.

- How intense is the lower back pain?
- Do you have difficulty in sleeping?
- How difficult is to take care of yourself?
- How difficult is to stand on your feet < 1h?
- How difficult is to sit on a chair <1h?
- How difficult is to walk <1h?
- How difficult is to lift something?
- How difficult is to travel?
- How difficult is to drive a car <1h?
- How your social life was influenced?

The resulted score is the investigated parameter. Depending on the final score we determine the patient's disability to perform certain activities and the final score falls within a described intervals: 0-20 points then there is a minimum disability, 21-40 points there is a moderate disability, 41-50 points represents a major disability and bed rest is needed.

1.3. Consumed daily calories

The daily activity parameter refers to the calories needed by the patient to perform his daily living activities. It is computed using formulas derived from WHO estimation of metabolic rate [11] and it depends upon the gender and daily activity of the patient.

Parameter P represents the weight of the patient and parameter T represents the height of the patient.

Table 1. Recommended loss of daily calories (P is the weight of the patient and T is the height of the patient)

Age	Male (calories/day)	Female (calories/day)
10-18	16.6P + 77T + 572	7.4P + 482T + 217
18-30	15.4P – 27T + 717	13.3P + 334T +35
30-60	11.3P + 16 T + 901	8.7P – 25T + 865
above 60	8.8P + 1128T - 1071	9.2P + 637T – 321

2. The inference system

When a patient describes it's symptom he describes it using a degree of uncertainty. This uncertainty can be implemented in software systems using fuzzy inference system. Fuzzy logic extends the classical Boolean logic by introducing a degree of uncertainty. The two major parts of a fuzzy inference system (FIS) are the linguistic variables which map precise numerical data in vague linguistic data and the inference rules which infer a result. The used inference system is a Sugeno type inference system [12] because the system returns three possibilities: operation, medical treatment and healthy patient.

2.1. Linguistic variables

In our case we used seven linguistic variables. Two of the variables describe the demographic data of the patients described by the sex and age, two variables describe the quality of life by the mean of the pain questionnaire and the consumed calories and the rest describe the range of motion measured with the ZM. They are constructed according to the following list:

- *SEX: MALE – FEMALE* represented by singletons;
- *AGE: TEEN* 10-18, *YOUNG* 17-32, *ADULT* 30-60, *OLD* 58-100;
- *PAIN:* 0-20 *LOW*, 18-40 *MEDIUM*, 38-50 *HIGH*;
- *CALORIES*: 1500-1800 *LOW*, 1700-2500 *NORMAL*, 2400-4000 *HIGH*;
- *FLEXION*: 60-80 *LOW*, 78-92 *NORMAL*, 90-100 *HIGH*;
- *EXTENSION*: 10-20 *LOW*, 18-30 *NORMAL*, 28-40 *HIGH;*
- *ROTATION*: 15-30 *LOW*, 28-45 *NORMAL*, 43-60 *HIGH*;

Except for the sex each linguistic variable is constructed using trapezoidal membership functions.

2.2. Inference rules

These rules are similar to the natural language communication. In their general form the rules are constructed by using antecedents and results separated by the "THEN" statement. The antecedent is a conjunction of several fuzzy terms logical operators.

The antecedents of the rules are the collected clinical data and the result of the rules is a suggestion to perform or not spinal cord correction surgery. In our case 243 rules were computed. 51 of the rules send the patient to operation and 159 rules indicates the need of medical recovery by treatment and 33 rules indicates a healthy patient.

3. Initial results and conclusions

The first test of the system was realized using a group of 15 control patients how have been already diagnosed. All patients are adults, 8 male and 7 female patients with divers' numerical results. To determine if the FIS works correctly we have analysed the same group and compared the results. The results are presented in Figure 1.

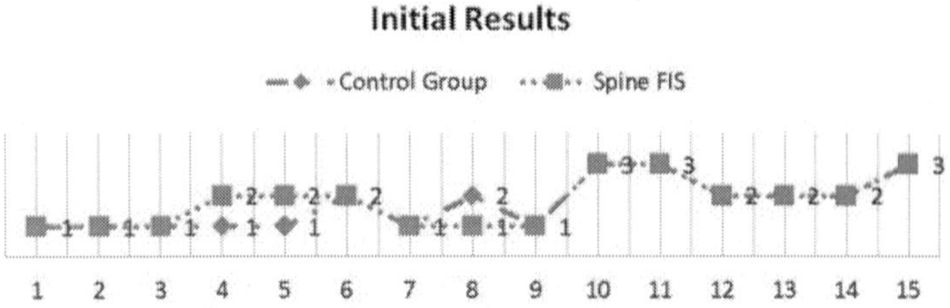

Figure 1. Initial results of the SpineFIS system, Results: 1-surgery, 2-medication, 3-healthy patient

In two situations, the FIS suggested that the medical recovery is preferred over surgery and in one situation suggested surgery over medical recovery. This difference is acceptable because 65% of the rules suggest medical recovery and only 21% of the rules suggest surgery. There is correlation of 0.83 between the results of the control group and the results of the SpineFIS.

The system has the ability to identify the correct treatment and can ensure the quality of the treatment. The patient will follow a correct and rapid treatment, which allows a quick return to an independent and fulfilling life.

References

[1] I. Halbert et al, *Proc. Natl. Acad Sci.*, USA, 1996, 9748.

[2] C.M. Herbert, K.A. Lindberg, I. Jaysonivi, A.J. Bailey, Proceedings: Intervertebral disc collagen in degenerative disc disease, *Ann Rheum Dis*, **34**(5) (1975), 467-68.

[3] D.G. Borenstein. - Epidemiology, etiology, diagnostic evaluation, and treatment of low back pain, *Curr Opin Rheumatol* **9** (1997), 144-50.

[4] F. Fitzpatrick, E.M. Badley, An overview of disability, *B J Rheumatol*, **35** (1996), 184-187.

[5] A.A. Guccione, A.M. Jette, Assessing limitations in physical function in patients with arthritis, *Arthritis Care Res* **1** (1988), 170-176.

[6] F. Guillemin, Functional disability and quality-of-life assessment in clinical practice, *Rheumatology (Oxford)* **39** Suppl 1 (2000), 17-23

[7] B.H. Guiot, R.G. Fessler, Molecular Biology of degenerative disc disease, *Neurosurg* **47**(5) (2000), 1034-1036.

[8] http://www.scientificspine.com/spine-scores/oswestry-disabilityindex.html (Accessed: 2013-10-16).

[9] http://www.tac.vic.gov.au/media/upload/quebec_scale.pdf, (Accessed: 2013-10-17).

[10] M. Toth-Tascau D.I. Stoia, D. Andrei, Integrated methodology for a future expert system used in low back pain management, *Applied Computational Intelligence and Informatics (SACI), 2012 7th IEEE International Symposium on* (2012), 315-320.

[11] Human energy requirements: Energy Requirement of Adults, *Report of a Joint FAO/WHO/UNU Expert Consultation*. Food and Agriculture Organization of the United Nations, (Accessed 2013-10-1).

[12] E. Araujo, Improved Takagi-Sugeno fuzzy approach, *Fuzzy Systems,* (2008) 1154 – 1158.

L. Stoicu-Tivadar et al. (Eds.)

doi:10.3233/978-1-61499-389-6-53

Preclinical tests of an Android Based Dietary Logging Application

István KÓSA[a,b,1], István VASSÁNYI[a], Balázs PINTÉR[a], Márta NEMES[a], Krisztina KÁMÁNNÉ[b] and László KOHUT[b]
[a]*Medical Informatics R&D Center, University of Pannonia, Hungary*
[b]*Cardiac Rehabilitation Centre of Military Hospital, Balatonfüred, Hungary*

Abstract. The paper describes the first, preclinical evaluation of a dietary logging application developed at the University of Pannonia, Hungary. The mobile user interface is briefly introduced. The three evaluation phases examined the completeness and contents of the dietary database and the time expenditure of the mobile based diet logging procedure. The results show that although there are substantial individual differences between various dietary databases, the expectable difference with respect to nutrient contents is below 10% on typical institutional menu list. Another important finding is that the time needed to record the meals can be reduced to about 3 minutes daily especially if the user uses set-based search. Conclusion: a well designed user interface on a mobile device is a viable and reliable way for a personalized lifestyle support service.

Keywords. Health monitoring, Diet coaching, Life style counseling.

1. Introduction

Most of the so called civilisation illnesses root in deviations from the proper life style. The correction of these deviations is a human effort intensive procedure, but modern info-communication tools can support some steps of this task. The use of a life style mirror application for dietary counseling is a typical function, where apps of mobile devices can be very effective. In order to prepare a personalized dietary analysis, one needs a reliable dietary log. The basis of most computerized services available for dietary logging is a Food Composition Database (FCDB) with the nutrient content for a wide range of common foods. Nutrients are the basic carbohydrates, proteins, minerals, vitamins etc. and foods are either ingredients of dishes (like white flour or olive oil) or they are consumed alone like apple or red wine. Some FCDB's, like the USDA SR FCDB are free for download [1]. In order to compute the nutrient content of the user's meals, the dietary database must also contain a highly culture-specific set of recipes as well. Several web-based or mobile applications support the logging of the user's meal and other services like daily/weekly overview charts, support for losing or gaining weight etc. The Calorie Counter android application boasts with the biggest recipe database of more than half a million [2], a large part of which was contributed by the users. Similar applications, with a smaller database, are the My Diet Diary and Tracker 2 Go [3, 4].

[1] Corresponding Author.

Though such services provide detailed nutritional analysis, the accuracy attainable by such FCDB-based systems was seldom evaluated [5, 6].

2. Purpose

The purpose of the current, preclinical study was to evaluate the capabilities of Lavinia life style mirror application and food composition database regarding the completeness and contents of the database and the time consumption of the logging procedure based on real life data of a medical institution in Hungary.

3. Overview of the Lavinia logging application

The Lavinia dietary logging application was developed at the Medical Informatics R&D Centre at the University of Pannonia, Veszprem, Hungary, to support dietary logging on mobile interfaces, dietary log analysis, and personalized menu generation using a dietary database specialized for the Hungarian culture. Its database currently stores 9500 food items along with their nutrient contents and 1373 dishes composed from the foods, but on the android user interface, we show only the most important 299 dishes and 360 foods, organized in 195 sets, to simplify the search and thus preserve user motivation. The system supports a hierarchical set-based search (see Fig. 1) as well as the usual keyword based search. We also allow to log generalized dish sets (like 'pasta') when the user does not find an exact match. If such a set is logged, we use the averaged nutrient contents of the set members in the analysis.

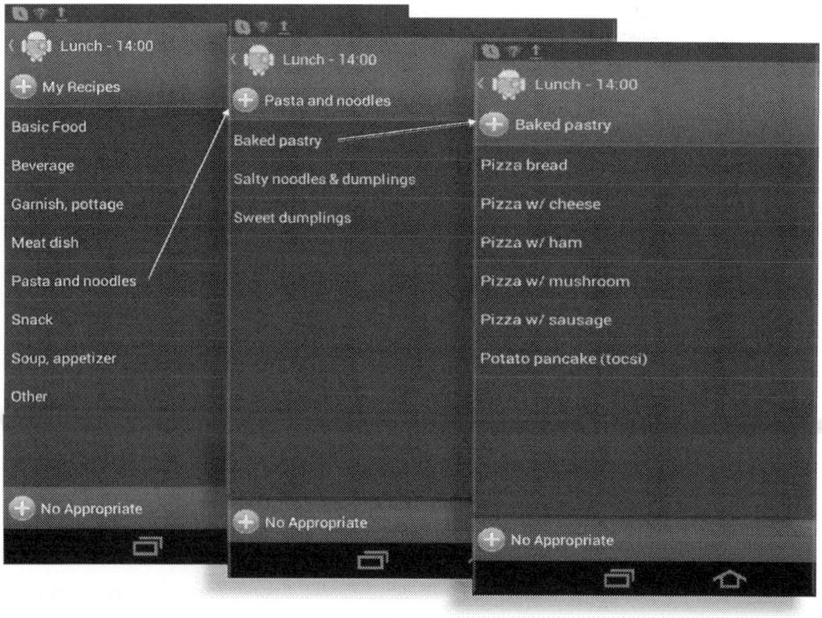

Figure 1. Screen shots of a set-based search procedure in the Lavinia mobile application

4. Methods

This study was performed using the dietary data of a medical institution, the Cardiac Rehabilitation Centre of the Military Hospital, Balatonfüred, Hungary. In the current, preclinical phase, only staff members were included to perform a final test before the planned clinical test of the system, in which typical patients treated in the institution will take part. The test period was 22 days long, for five different, manually compiled regular hospital menus, so in total we processed the meals for 110 days, with three meals per day, with Lavinia. The full list contained 1179 logged items with 156 different dishes and 38 foods (total 194). Some items occurred quite frequently, but there were also dishes specifically designed for a certain diet. For the analysis, we had access to the nutrient contents computed manually by the dieticians of the hospital using official FCDB tables. The study comprised three distinct phases as follows.

4.1. Phase I

In this phase, we tested the completeness of the Lavinia database. For each food or dish item, we distinguished three cases: present in Lavinia with the same name, present but with another name ('hard-to-find' items), or missing. We computed the ratio of these three groups within the 194 distinct items and within the full list of 1179 items (referred to later as 'weighed' ratios), separately for foods and dishes.

4.2. Phase II

In this phase, the nutrient content of the Lavinia database was evaluated based on all food and recipe types that occurred in the menus. As a preparation, we entered all items into the Lavinia database, that were identified as missing in Phase I, using publicly available recipes. To make the nutrient contents comparison possible, we first normalised the serving units of the items to match the units in the Lavinia system. Then two dieticians of the two institutions compared the most important nutrient contents (carbohydrates, protein and fat) computed by Lavinia and the hospital system, and labelled each differing case with consensus as due to 1) natural FCDB differences, 2) user search error, or 3) FCDB or system error. For the first group of cases, we then selected those items that had a nutrient content above 10 g. The amount of nutrients of the selected items was compared using Lavinia and the hospital system. Differences were expressed as absolute (g) as well as relative values (percentage of amount in the Lavinia system). Average differences as well as standard deviations of the differences for all nutrient types were calculated.

4.3. Phase III

The time expenditure of the mobile based logging procedure was measured using the same hospital menu set with 1179 items as used for previous studies. Five persons, familiar with mobile phone usage, but new to our set based dietary logging user interface received a short (3 to 5 minutes) introduction to the operations in the Lavinia system. Then they entered the list in the Lavinia system. The activity of the test subjects was logged and time stamped by the application from the start of any new item entry to the completion of the process. The switch from the set based search to the free text based search was allowed at any point for the subjects. We measured the average time spent for an item at the beginning and end of the process. The application start up time was not considered, assuming continuous stand by position for the investigated application in the background on the android system.

5. Results and discussion

5.1. Phase I

Considering foods and dishes together, 68% of them were supported with the same name, 7.7% with a different name, and 24.2% were missing. The missing items, however, were mostly special ones occurring rarely. For this reason, the 'weighed' ratios were better: 86.8% (same name), 4.1% (different name) and only 9.2% (missing), a more encouraging result. Considering only dishes, 66.0% (weighed: 79.2%) were supported with the same name, 7.7% (weighed: 4.8%) with a different name and 26.3% (weighed: 16.0%) were missing, the latter mainly due to special dishes designed for diabetic patients. For the foods only, 76.3% (weighed: 93.1%) of them were supported with the same name, 7.9% (weighed: 3.4%) with a different name and only 15.8% (weighed: 3.4%) were missing. As a conclusion from the user's perspective, we can roughly say that the chance of not finding an item is around 15%. Although for such a dietary logging application the food and dish search list can be infinitively expanded, we must spare the user's time (see Phase III results), so this ratio is highly acceptable.

5.2. Phases II and III

The nutrient content differences were considered natural FCDB differences (type 1 error) for 172 foods/dishes, while user search (type 2) error occurred in 11 cases. In the remaining 11 (type 3) cases, 4 items were erroneously recorded in the hospital system, other 4 in the Lavinia database, and in three cases a computation error occurred due to sets being chosen instead of exact items. The effect of natural FCDB differences was evaluated based on the 172 type 1 cases. The results are summarised in Table 1 for the three most important energy nutrients. The results show that although there are substantial individual differences, the expectable (averaged) difference is below 10%.

Table 1. Absolute and relative differences between the nutrient contents calculated by Lavinia and the hospital databases. Only those items were considered that contained at least 10 g of the nutrient.

Nutrient	No. of items	Avg. content [g]	Avg. abs. diff. [g]	Avg. rel. diff. [%]
CH	95	28.11 ± 18.67	2.49 ± 9,02	7.60 ± 35.89
Protein	67	18.91 ± 7.45	1.16 ± 4.93	5.13 ± 28.54
Fat	79	18.32 ± 6.73	2.47 ± 7.17	9.53 ± 37.47

This study analysed the inevitable differences and errors in food composition databases, an often overlooked issue in dietary analysis. There are other types of errors that occur in nutritional logging, but the proper management of this error is imperative when building a complex logging system including nutritional, workout and drug utilisation data.

In Phase III, five persons recorded the institutional menus in Lavinia for the investigated 22 days with an average of 12.0 items per day. The average net time consumption for entering a single item decreased considerably from 25.60 sec on the first day to 12.45 sec on the last, with a typical logarithmical learning curve ($time =$

$-4.06 \cdot \ln days + 26.95$). This decrease was dominated by the acceleration of the set based recording from 24.89 sec to 12.00 sec ($time = -3.52 \cdot \ln days + 22.71, R2 = 0.75$), while neither the frequency nor the time consumption of keyword based search was changed during this short period (13.4%, extra 22.15 sec.). The overall result is that the average total daily time consumption of dietary logging decreased from 6.80 min to 2.61 min ($time = -0.86 \cdot \ln days + 5.49, R2 = 0.65$). The ca. three minutes daily time consumption is quite satisfactory and justifies the simple mobile phone based dietary logging approach over other alternatives [6].

6. Conclusions

A general conclusion is that although single items in the Lavinia dietary log may be missing or quite inaccurate with respect to nutrient content, the summed resultant of these positive/negative errors is quite low for a longer period. The studies presented show that a relatively simple database with a well designed user interface can deliver a nutrient estimation at an acceptable time expenditure, which can be the base of more complex patient management systems.

The attitude of typical patients having undergone cardiac rehabilitation treatment can be evaluated after the completion of our planned clinical trials, which are currently under ethical consideration.

Acknowledgement

The work presented was supported by the European Union and co-funded by the European Social Fund, project title: "Telemedicine-focused research activities in the field of Mathematics, Informatics and Medical Sciences", project number: TÁMOP-4.2.2.A-11/1/KONV-2012-0073.

References

[1] USDA National Nutrient Database. http://www.ars.usda.gov/main/main.htm. (verified Mar. 2014).
[2] Caloric Counter PRO MyNetDiary (verified Sept. 2013) https://play.google.com/store/apps/details?id=com.fourtechnologies.mynetdiary.ad .
[3] My Diet Diary. (verified Sept. 2013) https://play.google.com/store/apps/details?id=org.medhelp.mydiet .
[4] Tracker 2 Go. (verified Sept. 2013) https://play.google.com/store/apps/details?id=com.byoni.tracker2go .
[5] G. Deharveng, U.R. Charrondiere, N. Slimani, D.A. Southgate, E. Riboli, Comparison of nutrients in the food composition tables available in the nine European countries participating in EPIC, European Prospective Investigation into Cancer and Nutrition. *Eur J Clin Nutr* **53** (1999), 60-79.
[6] P. Hakala, L.R. Knuts, A. Vuorinen, N. Hammar, W. Becker, Comparison of nutrient intake data calculated on the basis of two different databases, Results and experiences from a Swedish-Finnish study.*Eur J Clin Nutr* **57** (2003), 1035-1044.
[7] Vassanyi et al., Dietary Logging and Analysis for Tele-Care Using Harmony Rules. *Proc. Med-e-Tel'2013.* In Malina Jordanova (ed.) Global Telemedicine and eHealth Updates: Knowledge Resources", Vol. 6 (2013), 379-383.
[8] M. Rusin, E. Årsand, G. Hartvigsen, Functionalities and input methods for recording food intake: A systematic review, *International Journal of Medical Informatics* **82** (2013), 653–64.

Cross-Border Challenges in Informatics with a Focus on Disease Surveillance and Utilising Big Data
L. Stoicu-Tivadar et al. (Eds.)

doi:10.3233/978-1-61499-389-6-59

The Israel National Hospital Discharge Register: An Essential Component of Data Driven Healthcare

Ziona HAKLAI[a,1], Dmitry MOSTOVOY[a], Ethel-Sherry GORDON[a], Jean Chaim KARGER[a] and Assa REICHERT[b]
[a] *Health Information Division, Ministry of Health, Jerusalem, Israel*
[b] *Healsis Medical Technologies, Herzelia, Israel*

Abstract. The Israel National Hospital Discharge Register (INHDR) is an essential section of healthcare data. It includes record for each admission to hospital wards during the last twenty years, and the data are increasing by digitally updated information from hospitals on continually a monthly or quarterly basis. The register contains encrypted patient identity number, admission number, demographic and geographic data, hospitalization data, diagnoses, procedures and accounting data. The goal of the register is to measure medical and surgical services in hospitals, to compare hospital activity among regions, gender and age and population groups within the country and among other countries, to analyse the difference between periods. This large-scale hospital data helps in planning of the hospital services, analysing the health status of the population, disease and injury surveillance, and helps in performance of quality indicators. It assists decision makers at the Ministry of Health (MOH) in their daily and on-going missions.

Keywords. Hospital discharges, Hospital quality indicators, Information-driven healthcare, Big data.

Introduction

As standard healthcare moves to Evidence-Based Medicine (EBM) or Information-Driven Healthcare and to Patient-Centred Medicine (PCM) the concept of 4P Medicine - Preventive, Personalized, Predictive and Participatory is emerging [1]. The ultimate goal is to enable a more predictive, individualized, economical and safer healthcare by shifting from the evaluation of medical interventions in the average patient to the identification of the best intervention for each individual patient.

1. The Big Data Problem

To achieve the goals there is a need for the smart use of the ever-increasing amount of data available, both structured and unstructured, from multiple sources, and for tools for analysing the continual data streams produced for and by patients at every point of

[1] Corresponding Author.

care. This is referred to as the "big data" problem [2]. Big data should reduce the statistical errors, reduce the risks of mistakes driven from inter- and intra-seasonal and yearly fluctuations, identify rare healthcare phenomena, and allow for the discovery of patterns within smaller and smaller subgroups of patients and resulting in better predictions.

2. Israeli National Register

The key component of this work is the Israeli National Hospital Discharge Register (INHDR). The goal of this database is to measure hospital activity, to analyse trends and directions, and to document and quantify medical and surgical services etc. This capability gives the repository a great value in assisting decision makers at the Ministry of Health (MOH) in their daily missions. The repository is used regularly for policymaking and for the planning of services within the healthcare system. These large-scale hospital data sets are at the heart of the diagnostic and forecasting systems that make predictions regarding health status and outcomes for individuals and populations.

The INHDR is a 40GB database and is an output of the increasing use of electronic medical records systems (EMR) at hospitals. Maintaining an INHDR at the national level, with a high coverage rate, is a strategic issue for data-driven healthcare.

Hospital discharge data are a key element in solving many issues, among them are the following [3]:

- Healthcare Planning,
- Quality Assessment and Performance Improvement,
- Health Services and Health Policy Research,
- Injury Surveillance and Prevention,
- Disease Surveillance and Disease Registries Item.

Situated at the Israeli MOH, the enormous database is continually updated with hospitals providing the information digitally on a monthly or quarterly basis. All acute care hospitals (public and private) are included in the INHDR, as well as some of the psychiatric and long-term care facilities. The database contains records of each individual admission. Patient identity numbers are encrypted to allow follow-up studies while preventing identification of individuals and in order to protect the privacy of the patient. The database includes demographic and hospitalization data, as follows:

- Demographic data include age, gender, city code, as well as the patient's HMO,
- Hospitalization data include general information such as the type of admission (elective or urgent) and the type of discharge (home, transfer to other facility, left against medical advice, or died),
- Detailed information on the departmental level such as the date of admission and discharge from each department,
- Diagnoses listed and procedures performed in each department are coded according to the ICD9-CM,
- Accounting information for each hospitalization is provided - the payer as well as the tariffs charged for the hospitalization.

3. Examples of applications using the INHDR

3.1. Example for quality of healthcare and injury surveillance projects: Lower limb amputation rates among diabetics

The MOH undertakes data linkage projects to monitor the quality of healthcare in Israel in order to determine health policy in specific areas. These projects include processing and evaluating changes of post-operative clinical complications, re-admission and mortality. The projects are on-going in several areas such as colon surgeries, craniotomies, fractures of neck of femur and other indicators.

The Organization Economic Countries Development (OECD) and universal quality institutions consider non-traumatic lower limb amputation among patients with diabetes as a measure of quality of care. While this indicator uses inpatient data, the focus is on measuring the quality of non-hospital primary care.

Mortality and morbidity rates of diabetes have been decreasing over the past decade. Is the rate of amputation decreasing as well? Are there differences in the rate of amputation among different ethnic groups or in different geographic areas? These are the research questions.

The study is based on the INHDR in the MOH. During the study, we identified specific and age adjusted rates of diabetic inpatients that underwent lower limb amputation during the last decade.

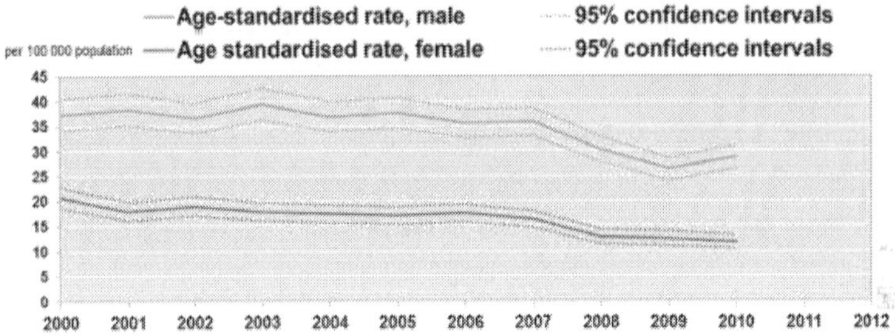

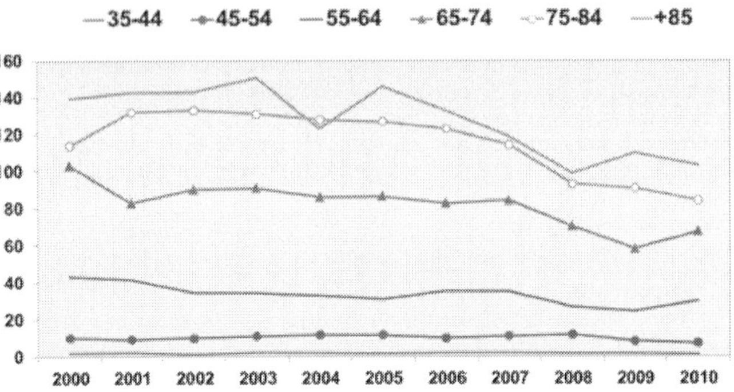

Figure 1 & 2. Lower Extremity Amputations in Diabetic Patients Rates per 100,000 persons.

Our findings show a steady decrease in the rates over the last 4 years. In addition, the age of the population undergoing amputation is steadily rising. This may reflect an improvement in diabetic care in the community and the utilization of a multidisciplinary approach when treating diabetic foot ulcers. There remains a large variance in the rates between population groups and different geographical areas within Israel.

As a conclusion we find these findings to raise the question whether this has to do with the quality of healthcare in these areas, i.e. the standard of care and access to care, or rather to the characteristics of the population in these areas, i.e. genetic heritage, diet, exercise, socioeconomic status and culture.

3.2. Example of use of the HDR for quality assessment and performance improvement: Readmissions to Internal Medicine Departments [4]

Hospital overcrowding is high in acute care departments in Israel compared with OECD countries, and overcrowding in internal medicine departments is particularly high. Research objective was to study the trends in readmission rates in internal medicine departments and to predict the risk factors for readmission.

The research is based on the INHDR. We analysed discharges from internal medicine departments that were admitted for at least two nights. Readmission was defined as overnight emergency admission within 30 days, with stays in internal medicine or ICU departments. Trends by demographic, hospitalization and morbidity characteristics are displayed. A multivariate regression analysis determined the risk factors for readmission adjusting for age, gender, surgical procedure, LOS, emergency, admission, diagnoses, and admission to ICU.

Results are the following. In 2011, there were 197 thousand hospitalizations discharged from internal medicine departments. The readmission rate was stable over the last decade, 19%-20%. The logistic model shows, patients with stays of 8 or more days have odds ratios (OR) to return within 30 days of 1.5 vs. patients with stays of 2-7 days. The risk for readmission increases with age (OR=1.7 for those aged 85 and over, 1.5 for those aged 75-84, and 1.4 for those aged 65-74, vs. those aged less than 65). Males have a higher risk (OR=1.2) vs. females. The OR for those with neoplasms was 1.7, with CHF was 1.5, and with renal failure 1.3 vs. those without these diseases.

As a conclusion, we can put that the rate of hospital readmissions in Israel was stable over the years. Health policy implications was to reduce the readmission rate through preventative treatment and continuity of care in the community, particularly for populations with co-morbidities to be coordinated with the health funds.

3.3. Example of use of the INHDR for Disease Surveillance: Kawasaki disease (KD) in Israel [5]

The study objective was to characterize the epidemiology and estimate the incidence of Kawasaki disease (KD) among children in Israel. By means of using the INHDR we investigated the epidemiologic features of KD among children less than 18 years of age between 1996 and 2009 in Israel. Incidence rates were calculated using the corresponding census data.

Results are the following. During 1996 through 2009, 685 children less than 18 years of age were hospitalized for KD in Israel. Eighty eight percent of these children were less than 5 years; the male/female ratio was 1.7 and most cases occurred in late winter-early spring. The overall incidence of KD was 6.4 per 100000 children less than 5 years of age. Since 2000, there was a gradual increase in KD incidence as well as an increase in the ratio of KD-associated hospitalizations to all-cause hospitalizations. For male patients under one year of age, rates of KD have almost doubled: from 5.8 per 100000 cases in 1996-1998 to an average of 11.9 cases per 100000 in the following years (p=0.002). The overall proportion of patients with coronary artery aneurysm (CAA) as a secondary discharge diagnosis was 2.9%, with higher rates of CAA among patients <1 or >5 years of age and in male patients.

As a conclusion, we can put that major epidemiologic features of KD among Israeli children are similar to those reported for the Caucasian population in Europe and the USA. KD incidence increased over the study period, especially among males less than 1 year of age. Higher rates of CAA among children <1 or >5 years of age warrant a higher index of suspicion for KD in these age groups. Continued surveillance for further rise in KD incidence in Israel is required.

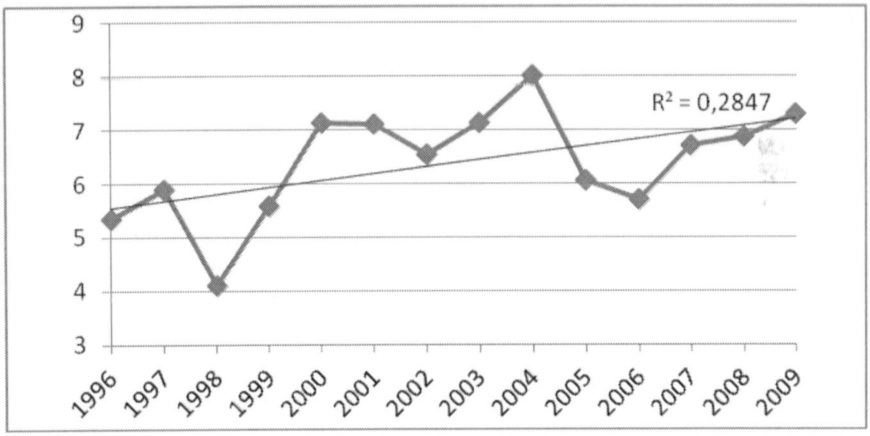

Figure 3. Annual incidence of KD in children < 5 years of age; rate per 100,000 children

4. Concluding remarks

This register is treasure of information that should be an essential component in all planning activities. The value of this treasure lies not with the cost of the register, but with its potential uses. Experiences at the Israeli Division of Health Information, with the INHDR show the usefulness of such a database for health research, especially during the lengthy period between the planning and implementation of a universal Electronic Health Record system.

References

[1] L. Hood, J.R. Heath, M.E. Phelps, B. Lin, Systems biology and new technologies enable predictive and preventative medicine, *Science,* **306** (2004), 640–643.

[2] J. Kyoungyoung, K. Gang-Hoon, Potentiality of Big Data in the Medical Sector: Focus on How to Reshape the Healthcare System, *Health Care Informatics Research* **19**(2) (2013).

[3] Schoenman, Julie. A, *The value of Hospital Discharges Databases*, Final report, 2005.

[4] S. Gordon Ethel, J. Meron, Z. Haklai, *Readmissions to Internal Medicine Departments*, MOH Israel.

[5] M. Bar-Meir, Z. Haklai, M. Dor, Kawasaki Disease in Israel, *Pediatr Infect Dis J*, **30**(7) (2011), 589-592.

Cross-Border Challenges in Informatics with a Focus on Disease Surveillance and Utilising Big Data 65
L. Stoicu-Tivadar et al. (Eds.)

doi:10.3233/978-1-61499-389-6-65

Supporting Diagnosis and Treatment in Medical Care Based on Big Data Processing

Oana-Sorina LUPŞE [a,1], Mihaela CRIŞAN-VIDA [a], Lăcrămioara STOICU-TIVADAR [a], and Elena BERNARD [b]
[a] *Department of Automation and Applied Informatics/University Politehnica Timişoara, Romania*
[b] *Department of Obstetrics and Gynecology/University of Medicine and Pharmacy "Victor Babeş", Timişoara, Romania*

Abstract With information and data in all domains growing every day, it is difficult to manage and extract useful knowledge for specific situations. This paper presents an integrated system architecture to support the activity in the Ob-Gin departments with further developments in using new technology to manage Big Data processing - using Google BigQuery - in the medical domain. The data collected and processed with Google BigQuery results from different sources: two Obstetrics & Gynaecology Departments, the TreatSuggest application - an application for suggesting treatments, and a home foetal surveillance system. Data is uploaded in Google BigQuery from Bega Hospital Timişoara, Romania. The analysed data is useful for the medical staff, researchers and statisticians from public health domain. The current work describes the technological architecture and its processing possibilities that in the future will be proved based on quality criteria to lead to a better decision process in diagnosis and public health.

Keywords. Healthcare Big Data, Cloud Computing, Google BigQuery, Treatments, HL7 CDA.

Introduction

We live in an era when people collect a lot of data and try to deal with it and use in different situations with maximum benefits. This led to a new term used when a lot of information is involved, Big Data. Big Data is a collection of large and complex data and information which is difficult to process with common database management tools. Big Data involve tools, processes and procedures that create, manipulate and manage very large data, and information in storage facilities. Four "V" dimensions describe the Big Data concept: volume, velocity, variability and veracity [1].

The healthcare domain is more and more based on the electronic medical record to store the patient's data and information about treatments and physicians. Using the electronic data makes it easier to access medical data, but the information grows bigger and bigger making difficult to draw useful conclusions from it without proper tools.

---

[1] Corresponding Author.

Day by day, the database of medical information is growing and the medical staff and big hospitals have difficulties to manage it. For this reason, the use of Big Data is very important in this domain. New technology will support the medical staff to manage information easier. Based on the suggested solution, which is a product of current work, information is inferred from complex heterogeneous patient sources. Correlations to the electronic health records of the patients are possible, large volumes of medical imaging data and extraction of useful information is easier, possibilities to analyse data and compare it with standard clinical data are provided, and also integration with data obtained from sensors located in the house of the patient [1].

The paper describes a case study of Big Data in healthcare, emphasizing the advantages of this technology in medical applications for collecting and processing data and extracting useful information for better treatments and surveillance of pregnant women. The Chapter 1 describes the software architecture of the Big Data system in healthcare with a practical approach in obstetrics & gynecology. The Chapter 2 presents Google BigQuery, a software tool from Google, which is useful for Big Data management, followed by the Conclusions reflecting the possibilities of technology use for the medical domain.

1. Big Data system architecture for healthcare

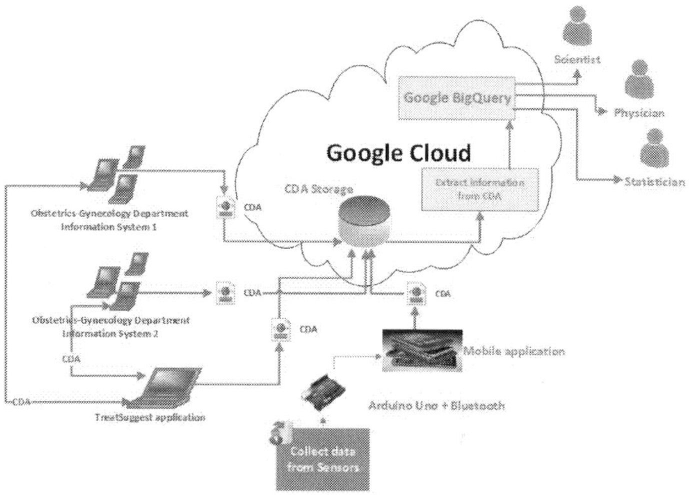

Figure 1. System Architecture

Figure 1 presents the system architecture with four components connected in a cloud, particularly Google Cloud, managing information about the patient. The components of the integrated system are:

- Two Obstetrics & Gynaecology Department Information Systems,
- The "TreatSuggest" application,
- A home fetal surveillance system that collects data from sensors and sends them to the cloud using Arduino Uno and Bluetooth,
- A mobile application. Communication between the components and in the cloud is using HL7 Clinical Document Architecture (HL7 CDA).

The Obstetrics & Gynecology Department Information System is an application developed in Visual Studio.NET 2010 using ASP.NET and C# language. The database is using Microsoft SQL Server 2008 [2]. The Obstetrics & Gynecology Department systems send a diagnostic and a treatment to the TreatSuggest application that will respond with a message if there is available a better treatment than the suggested one for a certain situation. The communication messages use HL7 CDA.

The component "TreatSuggest" is a medical application that supports physician's activity in selecting treatments for patients. The application is written in Visual Studio 2010, Visual C#. "TreatSuggest" suggests successful treatments and retrieves successful treatments from other physicians [3]. Physicians supply the information related to this component. All the successful treatments are saved in the local database of the physician and sent to a global treatments database. This justifies the necessity of involving the Big Data technology for processing. The "TreatSuggest" application is a local application that sends medical information about successful treatments in a cloud database and retrieves from it successful treatments for specific health conditions. The physicians may improve their work and increase the quality of the medical act dealing more easily with a big amount of data. The patients will receive better treatments based on evidence coming from peers on certain diseases. From the global database of treatments, using Big Data procedures, the treatments for a certain disease are extracted at the physician's request The database with the treatments contains the name of the disease, treatment for the disease previously input by peers of the domain and the characteristics of the patient. Data is not associated with personal information about the patient, so the security measures are the usual ones for this kind of applications. All the treatments are collected and analysed to obtain a better result for next treatments on other patients.

The fetal surveillance system component collects the data from the pregnant woman and sends it using an Arduino Uno component and a Bluetooth port to an Android application. The Android application creates an XML file - HL7 CDA standard and sends it to the cloud.

Communication between the systems and the cloud is based on HL7 CDA. This standard is a document mark-up standard that specifies the structure and semantics of "clinical documents" for the purpose of data exchange. It can include text, images, sounds, and other multimedia data and could be any of the following: discharge summary, referral, clinical summary, history/physical examination, diagnostic report, prescription, or public health report [4]. The information sent from the systems in the Google cloud is anonymous. It is not necessary to know the name and the personal ID of the patient because the Google BigQuery is used for statistical purposes supporting the work of physicians and researchers accessing the system. The security measures are the usual information systems ones, needing the name and the personal ID for identification in the system.

2. Using Google BigQuery

BigQuery is a web service based on RESTful, giving the possibility to analyse massively large datasets working in conjunction with Google Storage. Ii is an Infrastructure as a Service (IaaS) [5]. This web service ensures interactive analysis of up to billions of rows. It is scalable and easy to use, making developers possible to execute powerful data analytics on demand [6]. Several features of BigQuery are presented [5]:

- Data management (creates and deletes tables from different sources),
- Query (the queries are expressed in SQL language and the results are returned in JSON with a maximum reply length of approximately 64 MB),
- Integration (can use Google App Script, Google Spreadsheets or any language that can work with REST API),
- Access control (shares datasets with arbitrary individuals, groups, etc.).

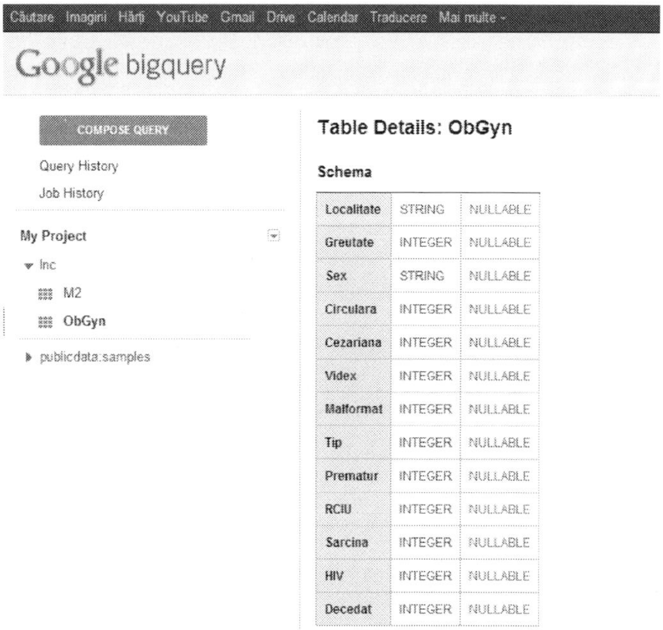

Figure 2. Data from the Obstetrics & Gynaecology Department information systems

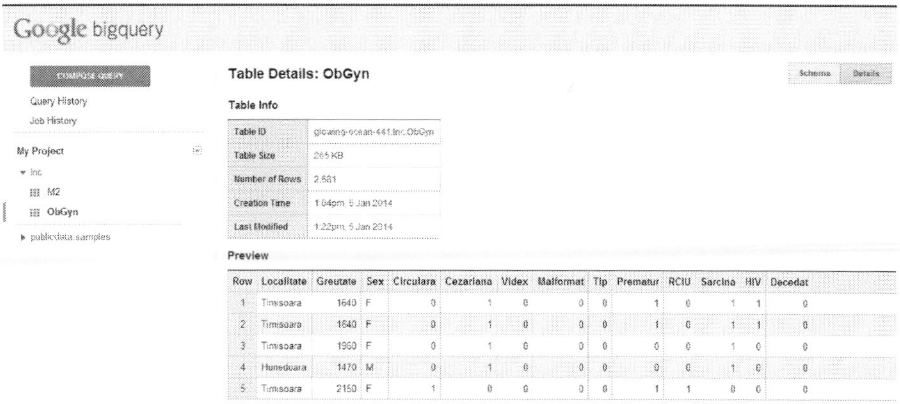

Figure 3. Medical data from ObGyn table

Google BiqQuery gives the possibility to analyse big amount of medical data received from different sources as a good solution for medical staff, researcher or statisticians. Figure 2 and Figure 3 present medical data uploaded in Google BigQuery that will be accessed with different tools supporting any language working with REST API, or Google App Script or Google Spreadsheets. The applications will send the information to Google cloud where will be stored. The stored information from Google cloud is used in BigQuery. The data is received in CDA format and on Google cloud will be available an application that extracts the needed data for the specific situation.

3. Conclusions

The paper presents a system architecture with integrated components: two Obstetrics-Gynaecology Department information systems, a treatment suggestion application and a home fetal surveillance application that sends medical information to Google cloud. The information is analysed using Google BiqQuery specialized in analysing big amount of data, responding to the medical staff need to analyse big amounts of data in the decision process.

The presented architecture and tools give a flexible frame for processing Big Data in order to obtain better results in patient treatment. Physicians have available an easy to use tool to obtain personalized diagnosis information for their patients. They describe in the system a particular situation and this is matched with the best result in the database in the cloud. The database is improving in real time with the results evaluated by the associated physicians. The processing is conveniently displayed as charts and graphics.

The work presented in this paper will be followed by proposing evaluation criteria for the solutions and parameters to validate the improvement in treatments.

References

[1] J. Sun, C. Reddy, Big Data Analytics for Healthcare, *Tutorial presentation at the SIAM International Conference on Data Mining*, Austin (2013).

[2] O. Lupşe, M. Vida, L. Stoicu-Tivadar, V. Stoicu-Tivadar, Using HL7 CDA and CCD standards to improve communication between healthcare information systems, *9th IEEE International Symposium on Intelligent Systems and Informatics, SISY, Serbia,* (2011), 435-457.

[3] O. Lupse, L. Stoicu-Tivadar, C. Golie, Assisted prescription based on successful treatments, *IEEE International Conference on e-Health and Bioengineering,* (2013).

[4] HL7 version 3 Interoperability Standards Normative Edition 2009, Based on HL7 v3 Data Types, Release 1, Disk 1 – Standards Publication

[5] Google BigQuery, http://en.wikipedia.org/wiki/BigQuery (accessed December 2014)

[6] Google BigQuery, https://developers.google.com/bigquery/ (accessed December 2014)

Cross-Border Challenges in Informatics with a Focus on Disease Surveillance and Utilising Big Data 71
L. Stoicu-Tivadar et al. (Eds.)

doi:10.3233/978-1-61499-389-6-71

From Generic Pathways to ICT-supported Horizontally Integrated Care: The SmartCare Approach and Convergence with Future Internet Assembly

Vladimir UROŠEVIĆ[a,1] and Marko MITIĆ[b]
[a]*Association for Medical Informatics of Serbia (AMIS)*
[b]*Belit Ltd., Serbia*

Abstract. Successful service integration in policy and practice requires both technology innovation and service process innovation being pursued and implemented at the same time. The SmartCare project (partially EC-funded under CIP ICT PSP Program) aims to achieve this through development, piloting and evaluation of ICT-based services, horizontally integrating health and social care in ten pilot regions, including Kraljevo region in Serbia. The project has identified and adopted two generic highest-level common thematic pathways in joint consolidation phase - integrated support for long-term care and integrated support after hospital discharge. A common set of standard functional specifications for an open ICT platform enabling the delivery of integrated care is being defined, around the challenges of data sharing, coordination and communication in these two formalized pathways. Implementation and system integration on technology and architecture level are to be based on open standards, multivendor interoperability, and leveraging on the current evolving open specification technology foundations developed in relevant projects across the European Research Area.

Keywords. Healthcare, Social care, Pathways, Services, Horizontal integration, Socio-technical Systems, Future Internet Infrastructures.

Introduction

The quest for horizontal integration of care delivery is in itself nothing new [1]. The approach aims at better joining-up of care services across established physical (regional, technological) or domain boundaries (social care and medical care, medicine and pharmacology) [2]. The SmartCare project (running from April 2013) pursues a dedicated program of service process innovation complemented by the development of ICT-based integrated care services, as experiences from earlier pilots suggest. The country sub-consortium for the Kraljevo pilot location in Serbia includes the local Social Work Centre, Health Centre, and Belit Ltd as the ICT service development and support provider.

[1] Corresponding Author.

1. The SmartCare Pilot Service approach

The policy and practice have fully recognised that fragmentation of care threatens quality and cost effectiveness [3]. The potential of ICT-enabled support could be exploited in a more effective way if they were not, as today, embedded in healthcare and social care services delivered in "silos".

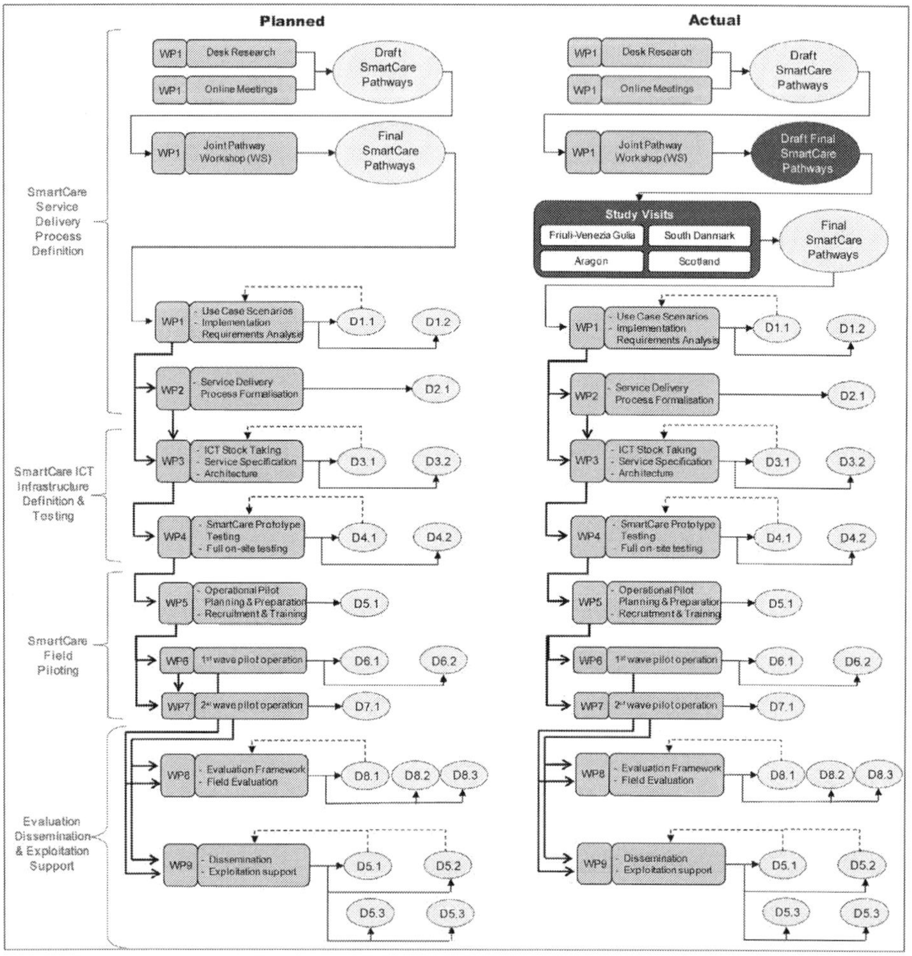

Figure 1. The extended SmartCare methodological approach

In a rigorous evaluation approach, the SmartCare pilots are to produce and document much needed evidence on the impact of integrated care, developing a common framework suitable for other regions in Europe, supporting long-term sustainability and up scaling of the services. The project has identified and confirmed two generic highest-level common thematic pathways in joint consolidation phase - integrated support for long-term care and integrated support after hospital discharge.

The sequencing of actions to be carried out, and the distribution of roles within each of the two confirmed generic highest-level common thematic pathways, largely varies, and horizontal integration of existing health and social care service practices across the 10 pilot regions comprises different levels of main activity:

- Joint work on the individual level when it comes to coupling up health care and social care around individual user in terms of case management and joint care teams.
- At the organisational level, new organisational structures and protocols are being put in place to tackle specific issues at the fault lines between health and social care.
- Finally, service integration tackles existing structural or policy barriers, primarily the funding of joint working practices, or strategic shift towards a more preventive agenda in health and social care.

In most pilot locations, except the most developed ones, the system of social care can be conveniently complemented, upgraded and enhanced with specific tools and add-ons following the models and structures of the usually more advanced healthcare IT systems, to implement and deploy the baseline interoperability on the level of common shared Integrated Care Records and Plans.

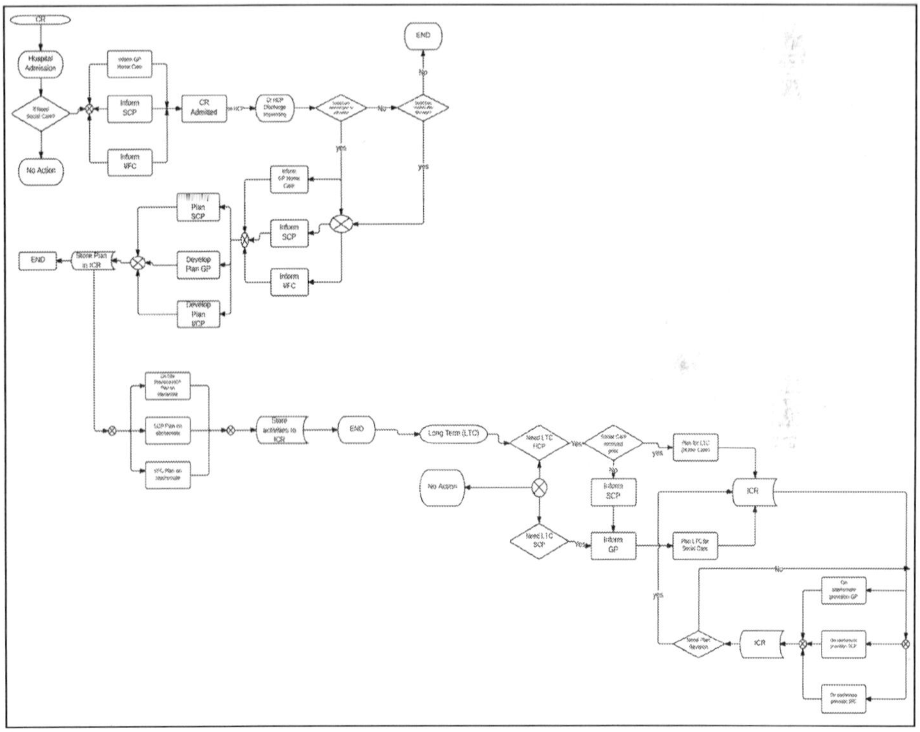

Figure 2. Tentative generic process model for main pathways on Serbia pilot location

Such is the case also in Kraljevo pilot location, with the social care IS being centralized and unified on national level distributed top-down, and health IT systems in primary and secondary HC developed and provided more rapidly through regulated competition and outsourcing from vendors, such as the PHC system jointly developed by Belit Ltd.

On locations such as South Denmark pilot, much more emphasis is on higher-level interoperability, tele-care, and multimedia data exchange [4].

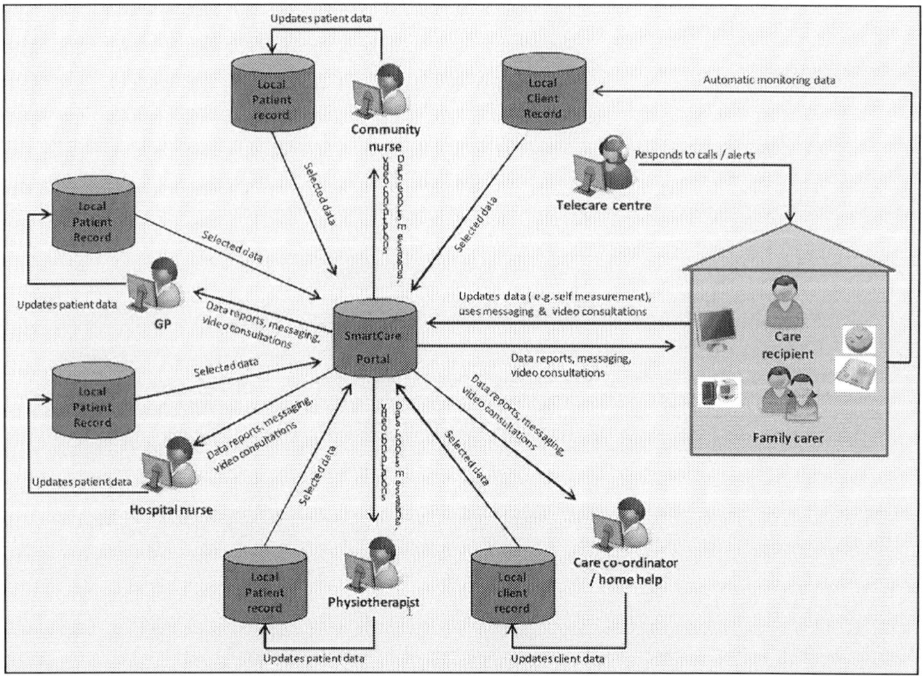

Figure 3. Schema of pilot service infrastructure implementation within the deployment context of South Denmark

2. Convergence and building on the Future Internet (FI) foundation

With implementation and system integration in the project aimed to be based on open standards and multivendor interoperability, a reasonable step further in architecture would be leveraging on the current cutting-edge and evolving open specification technology foundations and infrastructures developed in relevant projects and initiatives across the European Research Area, such as FI-PPP.

Envisaged complementarity between SmartCare as CIP project focused to field-implemented innovation and piloting, and a corresponding FI research project, such as ongoing FP7 FI-STAR in e-health, thus has high potential for reuse and wider adoption of the resulting services and tools.

3. Conclusion

In the Kraljevo pilot location, the development and specific implementation focuses on three specific objectives:

- Data integration and communication between the systems of healthcare and social work centres, improving the efficiency of staff teams and enabling access to system services also from mobile devices,
- Support for integrated care plans (ICPs) for all involved actors, including the necessary extensions of the systems in social work centres. ICPs are the

identified common and overlapping area between health and social care where workflow re-engineering can be performed. Care recipients themselves are also involved actors on provider side, in self-care use case scenarios. This implies also a needed module or set of generic services for facilitating and/or augmenting the use of advanced technology, as target CRs are mainly elderly or socially vulnerable category dependent persons with chronic conditions,
- Alerting, reminder and compliance tracking/verification services based on compiled integrated care plans, or just their scheduling data subsets, as inputs. The broadest generic range of reminders for appointments, therapy, social care interventions etc, and comprehensive verification/confirmation feedback types, such as audio/video/sensory, as outputs of the services, is intended to be covered, comprising the borderline scenarios (e.g. remotely observed therapy). These services will also comprise essential tele-care through monitoring cardiac parameters, with virtual devices in prototype.

In this aspect of higher target genericity, on wider level then being applicable in all project pilot locations, the considered implementation of developed services and components on the FI-WARE (General Enabler) paradigm has clear benefits on system architecture and technology levels.

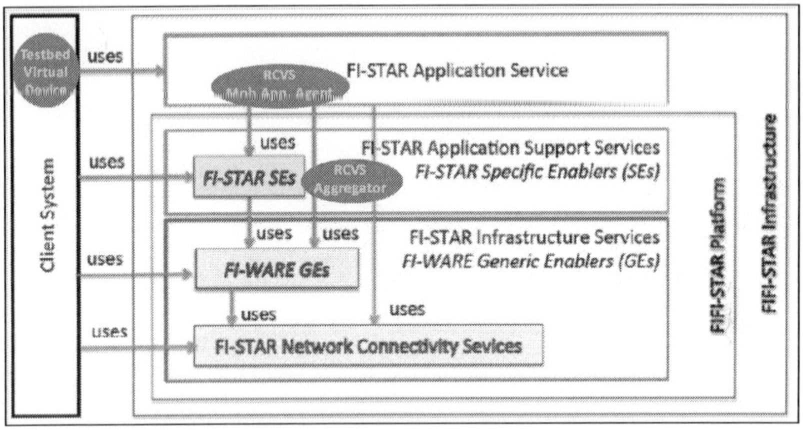

Figure 4. Conceptual Reminder and Compliance Verification Service (RCVS) components within the overall hi-level FI-STAR and FI-WARE platform architecture

References

[1] K.A. Stroetmann, L. Kubitschke, S. Robinson, V. Stroetmann, K. Cullen, D. McDaid, *How can telehealth help in the provision of integrated care?,* Policy brief 13, World Health Organization on behalf of the European Observatory on Health Systems and Policies, Copenhagen, 2010.

[2] K. Allen, J. Glasby, R. Rodrigues, *Joint working between Health and Social Care*, Long-term Care in Europe, Improving Policy and Practice, Macmillan, New York, 2013, 81-99.

[3] William A. Pasmore: *Designing Effective Organizations: The Sociotechnical Systems,* John Wiley & Sons, New York 1988.

[4] Jose Luis Mate and Andres Silva: *Requirements Engineering for Sociotechnical Systems* Information Science Publishing, Hershey, 2005.

L. Stoicu-Tivadar et al. (Eds.)

doi:10.3233/978-1-61499-389-6-77

Combined Model for Diabetes Lifestyle Support

Peter GYUK[a1], Istvan SZABO[a], Istvan VASSANYI[a], Istvan KOSA[a,b] and Levente KOVACS[c]
[a]*Medical Informatics R&D Center, University of Pannonia, Hungary*
[b]*Cardiac Rehabilitation Centre of Military Hospital, Balatonfüred, Hungary*
[c]*John von Neumann Faculty of Informatics, Obuda University, Budapest, Hungary*

Abstract. Treatment of diabetes mellitus is a public health related problem of modern healthcare. Surveys show that current methods to estimate the required amount of insulin are quite inefficient in practice as they are based on experience. This paper offers a new approach to predict the glucose level of people with diabetes. It combines two efficient models of the literature: one for nutrient absorption and one for glucose control. The combination of them tracks the blood sugar level considering nutrition composition, applied insulin and initial glucose level. Compared to already existing mixed meal models, the current version takes into account a more detailed nutrition composition (protein, lipid, monosaccharide, fiber and starch) supported by our expert dietary systems. Although the model gives satisfactory results even with parameter sets taken from literature, parameter training by genetic algorithms yields a better tracking of the patients.

Keywords. eHealth; Glucose-Insulin model; Glucose absorption; Diabetes

Introduction

Diabetes mellitus is a metabolic disease that affects our whole modern society. It is a typical disease of the modern culture mostly caused by obesity, the lack of physical activity and the changing of culinary culture. Currently, this problem hits 3% of the population [1]. Moreover, the number of the people with diabetes can reach 5% within some decades, according to current predictions [1]. This underlines the importance of diabetic lifestyle support.

In our work, we present a new approach to predict the glucose level of people with diabetes by combining a mixed meal model with a glucose-insulin one. We have focused on outpatients treated with insulin injections no matter having type 1 or type 2 diabetes [2]. For the insulin dose and timing, the patients normally use their own experience considering meals, physical activity, sports and the weather change. The main index to verify the patients' state is HbA_{1c} (Glycated hemoglobin). According to the recent surveys, these HbA_{1c} values are far from ideal in the case of most patients [3]. The gap does not seem big, but it can lead to serious complications.

The paper is structured as follows: Section 1 presents a short survey on related works. Section 2 includes the description of the proposed glucose level prediction system. Section 3 contains the result of several tests with the model, while Section 4

---

[1] Corresponding Author.

discusses the obtained results. Finally, Section 5 concludes the paper and outlines future work directions.

1. Short state-of-the art

The whole metabolism can be divided into two parts: nutrient absorption and glucose control. Our method is a combination of two existing models: one for glucose absorption and another for glucose modelling system including insulin evolution.

There are models for measuring glucose absorption from meals such as the Diabetes Advisory System (DIAS) [4]. This system operates with carbohydrate as input and takes some important components (e.g., lipids, proteins) out of consideration. Many models were built after DIAS, but their base is only a simple one-compartment model. The two-compartment model of [5] represents a more precise method by using Glycaemic Indices (GI) [6] in order to make simulations closer to reality.

The evolution of insulin is the other main factor in tracking glycaemia. There are also many methods in this field [7, 8] starting with the so-called minimal model [9]. Several methods approximate this model [10]. Methods that are more sophisticated use delayed-differential equations [11] to support subcutaneous insulin depot, create better representation of the Insulin Delivery Rate, etc.

2. The proposed method

A two-compartment method [5, 12] is often used to model the effect of nutrition to blood glucose level. The model proposed by T.Arleth et al. [5] divides the digestion into two segments (Figure 1). The food proceeds through the stomach compartment followed by the intestine, where the absorption of the monosaccharide happens. In contrast to simpler methods, this model takes protein, lipid, monosaccharide, fiber and starch as input, each one having its own effect during the absorption. Moreover, the method can deal with mixed meals by using GI, and digestion overlap is handled properly as well. The whole process is based on mass balance equations.

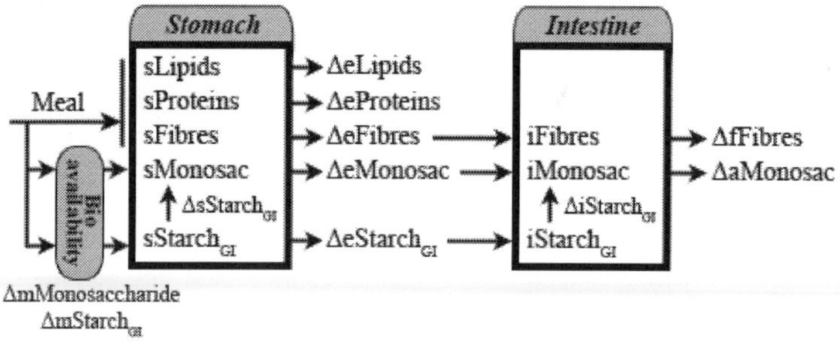

Figure 1. The process of absorption from mixed meals.

In order to model the glucose controlling process, the Delay Differential Equations (DDE) model has been chosen [12, 13]. In contrast to other methods (such as the minimal model) having a limited predictive power due to the low number of parameters, this model has several parameters supporting both type 1 and type 2 diabetics. It also allows insulin pump or subcutaneous insulin injections as input. The method uses two subcutaneous depots (accessible and not-accessible) to simulate subcutaneous insulin absorption.

The current article focuses on analysis, for further details of the models see [14].

2.1. The algorithm

To provide a better parameter set for the model, a genetic algorithm was used (Steady State Genetic Algorithm (SSGA) with jMetal framework [15]). The initial population consisted of the parameter set of the virtual patient from [14]. The fitness of a candidate parameter set was represented by an overall error rate computed from a Single Objective genetic algorithm creation [15].

3. Results

To validate the model obtained by the combination of the models highlighted in Section 2 and introduced in [14], as a first step we had done tests on virtual patients [16]. After that, two outpatients with diabetes mellitus were examined. The first patient was a woman with Type 2 diabetes (A), while the second test involved a Type 1 diabetic man (B). Both were treated with subcutaneous insulin injections, with similar protocols and the tests were executed with the same model parameters as with virtual patients.

Patient A was treated as inpatient to adjust her inordinate blood glucose levels. During the 6 days measurement, 15 meals and 45 glucose level values were logged; the latter was measured by an ordinary blood glucose meter. In the case of outpatient B, a controlled experiment was made during 3 days with 13 meals. To log blood sugar level, a Medtronic Guardian Real-Time Continuous Glucose Monitoring (CGM) System was used, measuring the actual value every 5 minutes.

Two different kinds of tests were made with each patient. The first simulation used meal wise records, i.e. the meals were treated as separate tests. Each test was run with zero start up blood insulin level and no running glucose absorption. The second test used a whole day's data for one day long test with zero start up blood insulin level in the morning. During this test, the absorption of the insulin and the glucose from food could be in progress at the next meal as well.

The change in the three parameters after the genetic algorithm was 78% in the case of patient A and 59% in the case of patient B.

Table 1. Comparison between the Two Tests with Patient A and Patient B

Patient A – 15 meals Patient B – 13 meals		Meal wise		Whole day		Whole day with genetic algorithm	
		A	B	A	B	A	B
Average deflection (mmol/l)		4.0	2.99	3.55	2.35	3.22	2.46
Error of prediction	< 3 mmol/l	50%	65%	61%	69%	61%	73%
	< 5 mmol/l	68%	76%	79%	81%	86%	77%
	< 8 mmol/l	93%	94%	93%	100%	96%	100%

4. Discussion

The results in Table 1 show that during the whole testing period better tracking results can obtained as it takes more factors into account. The model copes with insulin absorption and digestion overlap, which results in ca. 5% improvement of the error. The average error decreased by 0.5 mmol/l.

Comparing the two patients (see Figure 2), there is more than 1 mmol/l decrease in average error if the meals are more precisely logged. There is more than 10% increase in the error rate (<3mmol/l) that represents a significant improvement to any mixed meal model and protocol reported in the literature.

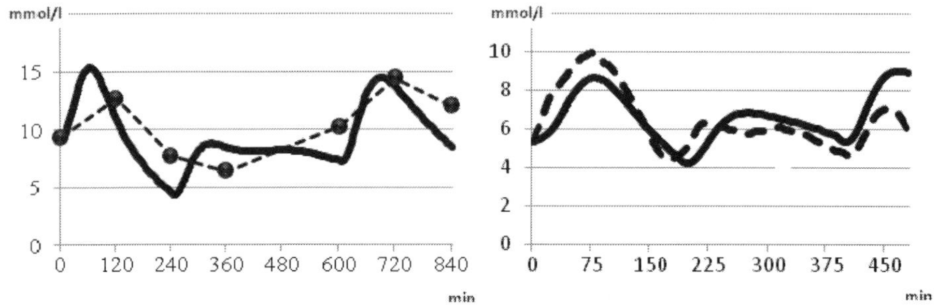

Figure 2. The fifth day of the meal wise test of patient A (left) and the first eight hours of the whole third day of patient B (right) (solid line – model estimations, dashed line – measured values)

We can also see that an ordinary blood sugar meter can lead to considerable errors in blood sugar level estimation. Analysing the meal wise test with patient A (Figure 2), it is noticeable that the patient measured a high value at 120 minutes, but the model shows even higher values between the two real-life measurements (0 min and 120 min). In this situation, the gap is small, but there could be bigger differences as well. The frequent presence of these situations can lead to higher HbA1c values.

In the case of genetic algorithm, the early tests (Table 1) show that there are more values under the margin of error (which is 3 mmol/l) for both patients with the new parameter set. This proves the need of control engineering methodologies and the efficiency of the genetic algorithm, even if it requires additional computational time.

5. Conclusion and future work

The paper presented a combined model-based approach for the short time prediction of the blood glucose level, based on the dietary log of diabetic patients. The results are satisfactory not needing any a priori identification protocol, but using genetic algorithms for model training. Further research is needed for:

- training the model to support personal variations in model parameters,
- extending the model to use also other physiological data available like physical activity and stress.

Our aim is to decrease the average error under one mmol/l, which is a significant and sufficient margin of error considering that the currently used real measurements have a similar margin of error. The results underline the importance of parameter identification. The model is currently evaluated in a clinical study with 20 rehabilitation patients as an add-on module to the specifically developed lifestyle mirror application (created at the University of Pannonia [17]). Our aim is to provide diabetics a dedicated mobile tool able to be used in their everyday life in order to predict their short time blood glucose levels.

Acknowledgement

The work presented was supported by the European Union and co-funded by the European Social Fund, project title: "Telemedicine-focused research activities in the field of Mathematics, Informatics and Medical Sciences", project number: TÁMOP-4.2.2.A-11/1/KONV-2012-0073. The János Bolyai Research Scholarship of the Hungarian Academy of Sciences and the GOP-1.1.1-11-2012-0055 project also supported Levente Kovács.

References

[1] S. Wild, G. Roglic, A. Green, R. Sicree, H. King, Global Prevalence of Diabetes: Estimates for the year 2000 and projections for 2030, *Diabetes Care* **27**(2004), 1047-1053.

[2] American Diabetes Association, Diagnosis and Classification of Diabetes Mellitus, *Diabetes Care* **27** (suppl 1) (2004), s5-s10.

[3] J. Nicholas, J. Charlton, A. Dregan, M.C. Gulliford, Recent HbA1c Values and Mortality Risk in Type 2 Diabetes. Population-Based Case-Control Study, *PLoS ONE* **8** (7) (2013), e68008, 1-7.

[4] S. Andreassen, O.K. Hejlesen, R. Hovorka, D.A. Cavan, *The diabetes advisory system – an IT approach to the management of insulin dependent diabetes*, in Brender J, Christensen JP, Scherrer JR, McNair P (eds.), *Medical Informatics Europe '96.* IOS Press, Amsterdam, Netherlands, (1996) 1079-1083.

[5] T. Arleth, S. Andreassen, M. Orsini-Federici, A. Timi, M. Massi-Benedetti, A model of glucose absorption from mixed meals. *In Proc. 4th IFAC Modelling and Control in Biomedical Systems Symposium* (2000), 307-312.

[6] D.J.A. Jenkins, T.M.S. Wolever, R.H. Taylor, H. Barker, H. Fielder, J.M. Baldwin, A.C. Bowling, H.C. Newman, A.L. Jenkins, Glycemic index of foods: a physiological basis for carbohydrates exchange. *American Journal of Clinical Nutrition*, **34** (1981) 362-366.

[7] Makroglou, J. Li, Y. Kuang, Mathematical models and software tools for the glucose-insulin regulatory system and diabetes: An overview, Applied Num. Math., **56** (3-4) (2006), 559-573.

[8] P. Palumbo, S. Ditlevsen, A. Bertuzzi, A. De Gaetano, Mathematical modeling of the glucose-insulin system: a review, *Mathematical Biosciences* **244** (2013), 69-81.

[9] R.N. Bergman, Y.Z. Ider, C.R. Bowden, C. Cobelli, Quantitative estimation of insulin sensitivity, *American Journal of Physiology*, **236** (1979), E667–E677.

[10] F. Chee, F. Tyrone, *Closed-loop control of blood glucose*. Springer-Verlag; Germany, 2007.

[11] P. Palumbo, P. Pepe, S. Panunzi, A. De Gaetano (2011). Glucose control by subcutaneous insulin administration: a DDE modelling approach, *In Proc. 18th IFAC World Congress*, Milan, Italy, (2011) 1471-1476.

[12] T. Arleth, S. Andreassen, M. Orsini-Federici, A. Timi, M. Massi-Benedetti (2005).Optimisation of a model of glucose absorption from mixed meals.(2005), 1-28.

[13] P. Palumbo, P. Pepe, S. Panunzi, A. De Gaetano, Observer-based glucose control via subcutaneous insulin administration, *In Proc. of IFAC Symposium of Biological and Medical Systems*, (2012), 107-12.

[14] I. Szabo, P. Gyuk, Lifestyle Log Based Blood Glucose Level Prediction for Outpatient Care. Accepted as full paper for *Int. Conf. eTELEMED*, Barcelona, Spain (2014).

[15] J.J. Durillo, A.J. Nebro, jMetal: a Java Framework for Multi-Objective Optimization. *Advances in Engineering Software*, **42** (2011), 760-771.

[16] S. Panunzi, A. De Gaetano, G. Mingrone, Advantages of the single delay model for the assessment of insulin sensitivity from the intravenous glucose tolerance test, *Theoretical Biology and Medical Modelling*, **7** (2010), 1-20.

[17] Pintér, I. Vassányi, B. Gaál, G. Kozmann, MenuGene: A Comprehensive Expert System for Dietary and Lifestyle Counseling and Tracking. *In Proc. 8th International Conference on Information Technology and Computer Science*, Athens, Greece (2012), 257-268.

Using Routine Data for Epidemiological Study and Public Health

L. Stoicu-Tivadar et al. (Eds.)

doi:10.3233/978-1-61499-389-6-85

Belgian Primary Care EPR: Assessment of Nationwide Routine Data Extraction

Etienne DE CLERCQ[a1], Viviane van CASTEREN[b], Nathalie BOSSUYT[b], Geert GODERIS[c] and Sarah MOREELS[b]
[a] *Research Institute for Health and Society (IRSS), UCL, Belgium*
[b] *Scientific Institute of Public Health (IPH), Unit of Epidemiology, Brussels, Belgium*
[c] *Academisch Centrum voor Huisartsgeneeskunde, KU Leuven, Belgium*

Abstract. Starting in 2009, the first ever Belgian nationwide data collection network using routine data extracted from primary care EPR (upload method) has been built from scratch. The network also uses a manual web-based data collection method. This paper compares these two methods by analysing missing and most recent values for certain parameters. We collected data from 4954 practices, pertaining to 29,180 patients. Mean values for the most recent parameters were similar regardless of which data collection method was used. Many missing recent values (>46%) were found for all of the parameters when using the upload method. It seems that, in Belgium, uploading routine data from primary care EPR on a large scale is suitable and allows the collection of chronological retrospective data. However, the method still requires major, carefully controlled improvements.

Keywords: Computerised Patient Record, Primary Healthcare, Data Collection.

Introduction

In 2009, the Belgian National Institute for Health and Disability Insurance (NIHDI) launched a complex intervention in primary care based on the chronic care model [1], called "care trajectories". As currently defined by the NIHDI, it organises and coordinates the treatment and follow-up for patients with Type 2 diabetes mellitus (DM-2) and chronic renal failure (CRF). The process starts with a contract being signed between the patient, the General Practitioner (GP), and a specialist.

Since 2009, the NIHDI has also funded the national ACHIL project (Ambulatory Care Health Information Laboratory), which assesses the quality of care delivered to patients covered by these care trajectories and monitors certain aspects of patients' health status (for instance HbA1c and eGFR) at an aggregated level.

Data collected for this project would ideally have been primarily extracted from GPs' EPR (Electronic Patient Records). However, using routinely collected general practice data for secondary usage (such as quality of care assessment), remains challenging [2-6]. Moreover, over 17 different software systems are currently being used by almost 10,000 practicing Belgian GPs, which hinders the rapid development of a secure primary care EPR-based research network.

---

[1] Corresponding Author.

This context has led the NIHDI to adopt a step-by-step approach. The first step (2009-2013) was to build a two-fold web-based data collection system that supports standardised forms for manual data capture as well as standardised data extraction from the EPR (upload). GPs can therefore freely choose their preferred method.

In this paper, we compare the two data collection methods and draw conclusions that should aid the future development of the national research network.

1. Methods

Recording patient data in the EPR and sending selected data to a research centre is foreseen by the care trajectory contract. The care trajectory program was started on 1 June 2009 for CRF patients and on 1 September 2009 for DM-2 patients.

Data was collected between May and September 2012 for all patients whose care trajectory began before 31 December 2011 and to cover a period starting the year prior to the start of their care trajectory and ending on 31 December 2011. Age and gender was collected for all patients. For DM-2 patients, additional data was collected relating to the following parameters: weight, height, systolic and diastolic blood pressure, LDL-cholesterol, and HbA1c. For CRF patients, additional data was collected relating to the following parameters: eGFR, systolic and diastolic blood pressure, PTH (parathormone), Hb (haemoglobinaemia), creatininaemia, and presence of Type 2 diabetes.

After identification and authentication, GPs connected to a specific web application hosted by a trusted third party (TTP) to send the data. GPs either entered patient data themselves or chose to extract the data from the EPR and upload it to the web application. The web application then performed validation tests (e.g. on data format and ranges). Following successful controls, an encrypted XML message was prepared for the research team that included only coded clinical data. Details of ACHIL privacy protection procedures have already been published [7].

In order to support the uploading procedure, each EPR software developer could decide to develop a specific extraction module, based on detailed specifications issued by the TTP in May 2012. Quality control of the extraction module had to be performed by the developers themselves. Additional data quality control procedures were applied at the research centre to control the entry of raw data (xml files) to the research database and to counter double entry of patients or parameters.

To compare the manual and upload data collection methods, we first report on the numbers of GPs, patients, contacts, and observations. We then analyse the number of missing values and the mean values for each parameter and outline some conclusions that may support the future development of the ACHIL network.

2. Results

We received usable data from 4954 practices, relating to 29,180 patients. This accounted for 77% of all patients involved in a care trajectory prior to 31 December 2011. Table 1 shows the basic figures for the research database. For technical reasons, in this paper, we discarded a small amount of data from a third data collection method called the “Réseau Santé Wallon”, which included 1353 care trajectory (CT) patients and 414 GPs. This did not affect our findings.

Table 1. Number of practices, patients, contacts, and observations by data collection method

Methods	Practices (N)	Patients (N)	Contacts (N)	Observations (N)
Manual	4600	26.444	40.203	199.057
Upload	354	2736	42.242	106.945
Total	4954	29.180	82.445	306.002

In Table 1, practices using both methods (1.03%) are counted twice. The percentages of patients that were registered twice, by different GPs or by different methods, were 0.77% and 0.20% respectively. In our database, 17,141 patients were enrolled in a DM-2 care trajectory (CT-DM2) and 12,629 patients were enrolled in a CRF care trajectory (CT-CRF). Two percent of these patients (590) were enrolled in both CTs. The median number of patients registered by practice (min: 1; max: 65) was four for the manual method and six for the upload method. For the manual method we found 1.31 observations by parameter and practice (mean value). This mean value rose to 7.4 for the upload method. Data was collected during a mean data collection period of 28 months. For both methods, the starting dates of the CTs were homogeneously spread over the entire observation period, with the exception of approximately 11% of the CTs using the upload method, which started on the first day of the official CT program. Figure 1 shows the contact registration dates by data collection method.

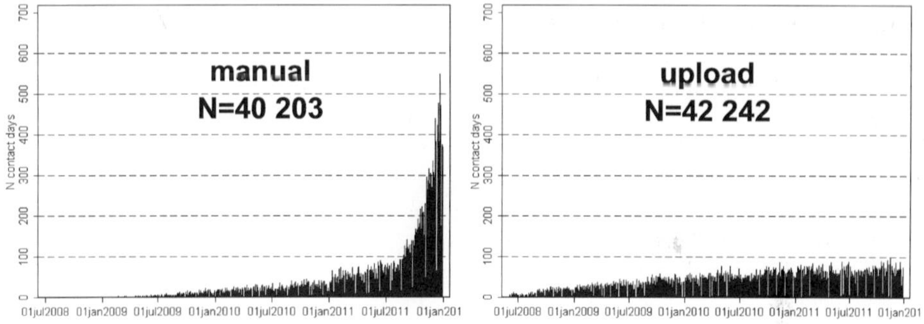

Figure 1. Number of contacts grouped by registration date and presented by registration method.

The mean age of the patients was 68 for CT-DM2 patients and 75 for CT-CRF patients, for both methods. Using the manual method, we found that 51.64% of CT-DM2 patients and 52.32% of CT-CRF patients were male and that 34.02% of CT-CRF patients were diabetic. Using the upload method, we found that 50.94% of CT-DM2 patients and 51.08% of CT-CRF patients were male and that only 5.31% of CT-CRF patients were diabetic.

Table 2 shows the numbers and percentages of missing most recent values for each parameter, by data collection method. Two time periods, one of four months and one of 12 months, were used to define recent values. For CT-DM2 patients, recent data (<4months) was missing for all the parameters for 25% of patients when using the manual method and for 12.94% of patients when using the upload method. These figures dropped to 4.90% and 2%, respectively, when a 12-month period was considered. For CT-CRF patients, recent data (<4months) was missing for all parameters for 27.90% of patients when using the manual method and for 19.15% of patients when using the upload method. These figures dropped to 9.10% and 5.56%, respectively, when a 12-month period was considered.

Table 2. Percentages of missing parameters, by data collection method and data collection period

DM-2 Care trajectory	Manual (N=15 541)		Upload (N=1600)		CRF Care trajectory	Manual (N=11 423)		Upload (N=1206)	
	missing <4 month	missing <12 month	missing <4 month	missing <12 month		missing <4 month	missing <12 month	missing <4 month	missing <12 month
HbA1c	29.19%	9.81%	57.81%	52.44%	eGFR*	32.50%	14.75%	61.44%	53.98%
LDL-chol.	35.17%	17.30%	80.31%	76.75%	Syst. BP	29.82%	11.52%	54.73%	48.92%
Syst. BP	27.08%	7.53%	52.81%	47.06%	Diast. BP	29.87%	11.61%	54.81%	49.25%
Diast. BP	27.12%	7.58%	52.88%	47.19%	PTH	58.25%	48.47%	89.14%	87.15%
BMI	35.72%	18.67%	73.81%	70.50%	Hb	37.35%	20.89%	62.35%	55.14%

* Calculated or registered eGFR; LDL-chol.: LDL-cholesterol; Syst. BP: Systolic blood pressure; Diast. BP: Diastolic blood pressure; BMI: Body Mass Index; PTH: Parathormone; Hb: Hemoglobinemia

Mean values of most recent parameters were similar regardless of which data collection method and data collection period were used. Hereafter, we will refer only to the figures for the manual data collection method and the 4-month data collection period. For CT-DM2 patients, mean values were: HbA1c: 7.51% (+/- 1.19); LDL-Cholesterol: 89.48 mg/dl (+/-33.63); systolic BP (blood pressure): 133.69 mmHg (+/- 14.91); diastolic BP: 77.82 mmHg (+/- 8.63), and BMI: 30.54 Kg/m² (+/-5.63). For CT-CRF patients the mean values were: registered eGFR: 31.17 ml/min.1.73m² (+/- 11.4); systolic BP: 133.55 mmHg (+/- 17.2); diastolic BP: 76.6 mmHg (+/- 9.39); PTH: 99.07 pg/dl (+/- 83.25), and Hb: 12.35 g/dl (+/- 1.83).

3. Discussion

Starting in 2009, it took almost three years to come up with an accepted network architecture that met an acceptable level of privacy protection [7]. Following this, only four months were left for the development of software extraction modules and data capture. Time was therefore lacking to set up a standardised quality control procedure for the extraction modules. Some GPs reported problems with installing these modules. At the TTP, a strong quality control procedure rejected all the messages without the correct format or with non-authorised values. GPs who had been using EPR for many years may have been reluctant to use a manual data collection procedure instead. All of this may partly explain why we did not receive any data for over 20% of the patients involved in a care trajectory and why 11% of patients started their care trajectory on the official start date of the care trajectory program, which was probably used by the software developers as “default” start date. However, confirmation of these hypotheses would require further investigations that have not yet been planned.

Our results clearly show that more contacts per patient and more observations by parameter were obtained when the upload method was used. This was even more obvious when missing data was taken into account. The upload method therefore seems more suited to obtaining chronological retrospective data.

Only 5.31% of CT-CRF patients were recognised as diabetic patients by the upload method. Based on previous results (using strong quality control procedures), some underestimation related to an EPR under-recording issue was expected (expected value around 24%) [5]. The current underestimation might therefore be largely related to the quality level of the extraction modules.

As expected, the number of missing most recent values decreased considerably when a 12-month data collection period was used. However, the number of missing most recent values was still unexpectedly high when the manual method was used. For example, using data from a national billing database (2010), we found that 97% of the

CT-DM2 patients had had their HbA1c measured in 2010. We found no indication of lower percentages in 2011. For the manual method, missing data could be partly explained by data being no longer available at GPs' offices (lab results having been given to the patients) or by a lack of communication between healthcare actors (lab tests having been ordered by another physician and the results not communicated to the treating GP). This, however, requires further investigation.

For the upload method, missing values for all of the parameters are unexpectedly high [5]. In addition to a well-known under-registration issue in the EPR [3-5], this could also be partly explained by low quality of the extraction modules.

It is also worth pointing out that patient profiles were similar, in terms of age, sex, and mean values of the various parameters, regardless of the method that was used.

4. Conclusions

Building research networks for health service management at a national scale raises issues not encountered by smaller pilot studies. Gaining the trust of the many different stakeholders is of the utmost importance and requires time and effort. Meanwhile, setting up rigorous standardised and centralised control procedures remains essential if the expected benefits are to be achieved. Currently, correctness of the extraction is still an issue but the national Belgian labelling programme of EPR software systems may help the required quality level to be achieved within the next two or three years.

Uploading data from EPR allows chronological retrospective data to be collected at a national scale. The use of manual data capture is definitely not an option.

In future, the properties of the research information network will evolve. The quality of the extraction modules will improve. More GPs will use the upload method for more patients, providing more data. There may also be improved data recording in the EPR and improved data communication between healthcare actors. We strongly suggest that such improvements of the properties of the research information network be measured and monitored, so that future changes in the quality of documented care, primarily for process parameters, may be interpreted.

This study was funded by the NIHDI.

References

[1] Wagner EH, Austin BT, Von Korff M. Organizing care for patients with chronic illness. Milbank Q 1996; 74(4):511-44

[2] de Lusignan S, Van Weel C. The use of routinely collected computer data for research in primary care: Opportunities and challenges. Fam Pract 2006; 23:253–63.

[3] Chan KS, Fowles JB, Weiner JP. Electronic Health Records and the Reliability and Validity of Quality Measures: A Review of the Literature. Med. Care Res. Rev. 2010; 67(5):503-27

[4] De Clercq E et al. Quality assessment of automatically extracted data from GPs' EPR. Stud Health Technol Inform, 2012, 180:726-30

[5] De Clercq E et al. Routinely-collected general practice data from the Electronic Patient Record and general practitioner active electronic questioning method: a comparative study. Stud Health Technol Inform, 2013; 192:510-4

[6] Pearce CM et al. The Computerized Medical Record as a Tool for Clinical Governance in Australian Primary Care. Interact J Med Res. 2013 Jul-Dec; 2(2):e26.

[7] De Clercq E et al.. Nation-Wide Primary Healthcare Research Network: a Privacy Protection Assessment. Stud Health Technol Inform 2012; 174:23-8.

Cross-Border Challenges in Informatics with a Focus on Disease Surveillance and Utilising Big Data 91
L. Stoicu-Tivadar et al. (Eds.)

doi:10.3233/978-1-61499-389-6-91

Improving Hospital Decision Making with Interpretable Associations over DataCubes

Carlos MOLINA [a,1], Belén PRADOS-SUAREZ [b], Miguel PRADOS DE REYES [c] and Carmen PEÑA YAÑEZ [b]
[a] *Department of Computer Sciences, University of Jaen, Jaen, Spain*
[b] *Department of Software Engineering, University of Granada, Granada, Spain*
[c] *Department of Computer Sciences, San Cecilio Hospital, Granada, Spain*

Abstract. In this paper we propose a new Classification based on Association Rules (CAR) algorithm that improves the interpretability of the results, works over real data from the electronic health records (EHRs), and allows the study of the patient as a whole. It enables tasks such as the discovery of relationships between diseases, or offering several alternative and reasoned diagnoses for the cases of patients with several diseases that analysed separately could lead to mistaken diagnosis. We aim to achieve several goals: to discover hidden relationships; to improve the interpretability and reduce the complexity of the result; to obtain more reliable diagnosis (getting alternative reasoned diagnoses and higher robustness to noisy rules), and to improve the quality of the classifier avoiding the usual over-fitting problem. To this purpose, we define and exploit hierarchies defined over datacubes dimensions, and change the way the association rules are obtained, and their evaluation at the classification process. To prove the utility of our proposal we have used it in an example of cancer discrimination.

Keywords. CAR, Complexity Reduction, Interpretability Improvement Classification, DataCube, Multidimensional Model.

Introduction

In the last few years important advances have been realized in the application of data mining methods over health care information with research purposes to improve the managerial decision support [1,2] or to support medical diagnosis [3,4].

Nevertheless as Jensen et al. indicate in [5], this is still an under-used source of information, due to three main reasons: the nature of the medical data itself; the use of statistical data instead of real data obtained directly from the electronic health records (EHR); and the difficulties for the user to understand and interpret the results of the data mining techniques. It all makes the medical doctors reluctant to the use of these advances, and especially the clinical decision support systems (CDSS) [6].

Here we propose a data mining method specifically designed to improve interpretability of the results that also works over real data. Therefore, although the proposal presented in this paper can be applied to any of these problems, here we focus on an example of use for CDSS.

[1] Corresponding Author.

Among the wide variety of data mining methods [7, 8] the most widely used on CDSS are the neural networks [9], the decision trees [10], or combinations of them [11]. The main inconvenience of these proposals is that they are specifically designed for concrete pathologies or parts of the human body. As Isola et al. states in [9], it is necessary to count on systems capable of analysing the medical data set as a whole, in order to find out interactions or relationships between pathologies or different diseases with similar symptoms for patients with several diseases whose symptoms may lead to confusion in the diagnosis, second opinions or alternative diagnosis.

With CAR proposals, it is possible to achieve these goals since, as it is well known [12], they are designed to discover relations, and in addition, they are the most precise techniques due to their exhaustive exploration of the possibilities. Nevertheless, they still have three inconveniences. First, their results are difficult to understand. This is due to the rule set obtained with CAR proposals, which is used as an ordered list of rules. This set is checked in order, discarding the rules unsatisfied and stopping the process at the first one satisfied. In real systems, the antecedents of these rules are usually complex and not directly meaningful, so the user must take into account the previously discarded rules to understand the full meaning of the classification performed. Second, they are not robust to noise, since they are based on the selection of a single response, so if the rule selected or any of the rules discarded are wrong the final response of the system will also be wrong. Finally, another problem that classification methods (not only CAR based) must face is the over-fitting of the data.

It is necessary to find techniques capable of working over real data from the EHRs, of finding out hidden relations, that are also robust to noise, offering a good classification without over-fitting, and that provide several and reasoned responses which must also be easy to understand. To achieve these goals we present our proposal, based on three key points: the use of "datacubes" and the exploitation of the hierarchies defined over their dimensions, the change in the way the association rules are obtained, and a change in the evaluation of the rules at the classification process.

In section 1, we show the adaptation of the algorithm to reduce the complexity of the resultant set of rules. Examples about the performance of our proposal are presented in section 2, and finally we indicate our conclusions and final remarks in section 3.

1. Algorithm

In this section, we present a modification of the Complexity Guided algorithm for Association Rule Extraction (COGARE) described in [13]. The modification proposed here aims to extract association rules adapted for classification. Next, we comment the changes that must be introduced.

Itemset generation. When generating the frequent itemsets we change the candidates and only consider the itemsets containing an item of the class variable. If the itemset is not frequent, the method applies the generalization process but not on the class item (the granularity of this variable does not change in any moment).

Rule generation. At the rule generation stage, the method only takes into account the association rules of the form A → C, where C only has one item that belongs to the class variable. Therefore, for each frequent itemset found, the method only generates one rule.

Rule generalization. In the rule generalization phase the scheme is similar to the itemset generation, because the method tries to generalize the rule set considering all the variables but the class.

Iterative approach. One of the main changes of the algorithm is the use of an iterative approach. Most of the proposals first generate all the association rules and later select the classification rules from this set. Here we propose the following iterative approach:

- First the method generates frequent itemsets of size 2 (one item from the class variable and another one from other variable),
- Then it generates the association rules of size two, pruning those with a certainty factor (CF) under the threshold given as parameter, and selects the rules from this set, so the method generates a classification model using simple rules (one antecedent and the class),
- Next, the method calculates the frequent itemset of size 3 using frequent itemsets of size 2. In this stage, the algorithm tries to reduce the number of rules, deleting unnecessary frequent itemsets as explained in the next subsection,
- After it the method generates the rules for the frequent itemsets of size 3, and selects the rules to classify,
- The method stops if the result is not better than using rules of size 2. If we obtain a better classification, the process continues with itemsets of size 4, and so on.

Space reduction. The aim of this process is to reduce the candidate frequent itemsets to be generated. The main idea is to avoid building more specific rules i.e. bigger itemsets in areas of the search space where the classification was made correctly with simpler rules. The method takes the current classification rule set, and looks for areas correctly classified with the current rule set. Those areas are delimited by the rules with CF equal to one (all the elements which satisfy the antecedent of the rule have the same class). Next, the process keeps out from the frequent itemsets those including the antecedent of any of these rules, and in the next iteration, no itemset in those areas will be considered. Avoiding the generation of larger and more complex rules in these areas, the use of unnecessary inserted items in the antecedent of the rules is also avoided, and hence the over-fitting they could introduce.

Rules selection. On each iteration, the algorithm selects a set of rules to build the classifier. First, the method sorts the rules according to the quality of each one in decreasing order (better rules first). Then it uses the first rule as initial classifier a computes its quality. The rest of the process checks iteratively whether the next rule improves the quality or not. If there is an improvement, the technique selects the rule and proceeds to the next iteration. Otherwise, the rule is dismissed.

Rule evaluation. As mentioned above in most of the CAR proposals the rule set obtained is used as an ordered list of rules. In our proposal, we do not establish an order between rules since we use a classic inference schema, considering that a rule is satisfied with a degree $\otimes(\mu(A_1), \ldots \mu(A_n))$, where A_is are the items in the antecedent and $\mu(Ai)$ the degree at which the record satisfies the item. As t-norm we use the *minimum*. We combine the result of each fired rule with the same consequent (class) with a t-conorm to obtain one unique value for each class (we use the *maximum*). The class with higher degree is the one selected to classify the new record.

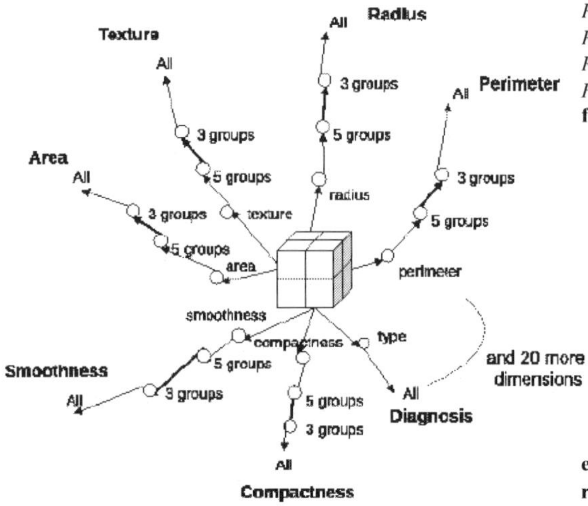

N = Number of variables
FI_2 = Generate frequent itemsets of size 2
R_2 = Generate rules from FI_2
R' = Sort R_2 according to rules quality
R_a = Selected rules from R'
FI_2 = reduceSpace(FI_2,R_a)
for i = 3 to N do
  FI_i = Generate frequent itemsets of size i from FI_{i-1}
  R_i = Generate rules from FI_i
  $R = \cup_{j=2}^{i} R_i$
  R' = Sort R according to rules quality
  R_c = Selected rule from R'
  if *Quality*(R_c) > *Quality*(R_a) then
    $R_a = R_c$
    FI_i=reduceSpace(FI_i,R_a)
  else
    Finish and *return* R_a
  end if
end for
return R_a

Figure 1. C_{Cancer} structure with Iterative process for rule generation

2. Example

To test the proposal we use the Wisconsin Diagnostic Breast Cancer (WDBC) at UCI ([14]). Features are computed from a digitized image of a fine needle aspirate (FNA) of a breast mass. They describe characteristics of the cell nuclei present in the image. We consider 31 attributes and a total of 569 instances. We build over each attribute a hierarchy with five values (*Very low, low, medium, high and very high*) and another with only three values (*low, medium and high*). To obtain the partition of the values into the categories we have used the method presented in [15]. With this datacube we want to know the estimated type of the cancer: *malignant* or *benign*, so we consider as class the dimension *Diagnosis*. The parameters for the process are the following: Support=0.005, CF=0.1, Max complexity=0.2 (value that sets a high reduction of the number of rules in the association rule extraction), AcceptRatio=1.2 (a worse rule set may be accepted if the complexity reduction is high), β=10 (penalty, in the generalization process, for using values which produce a rule set that was not accepted in the past), α=0.7 (having less rules is preferred to improving the abstraction). To test the quality of the method we apply 10-fold cross-validation getting and average correct classification of 95.129% with 47.7 rules on average. Therefore, the method gets a good result.

3. Conclusions

In this paper, we have presented a modification of the COGARE algorithm for the extraction of association rules. With the methodology proposed four goals, finding out hidden relations with the use of association rules may be achieved firstly. Secondly, we achieve robustness to noise, since we consider all the possible responses of the system, and provide the user with a combination of them too. Thirdly, an improvement of the interpretability of the results, since we have reduce the complexity of the result (less and simpler rules), and each rule is a result per se that can be interpreted independently. It means that each rule helps to understand not only the criteria under which the classification is being performed, but also the characteristics that determine each class. This research is still in progress and the algorithm is being tested under more data sets to be able to quantify the improvements in the above mentioned goals. Finally, we would like to remark that our proposal, which could also be applied for research purposes or managerial decision support, works over real data from the EHRs. It means that it can analyse the medical data set (and therefore the patient) as a whole, which is especially useful for tasks such as obtaining alternative diagnosis or discover relationships between diseases, offering also reasoning. It all may reduce the reservations of the medical doctors to use the CDSS.

References

[1] M. Nelson, R. Sen, Business rules management in healthcare: A lifecycle approach, *Decision Support Systems*, **57**, (2012), 387–394.

[2] N. Foshay, C. Kuziemsky, Towards an implementation framework for business intelligence in healthcare, *International Journal of Information Management*, **34**(1), 20-27, (2014).

[3] S. Ruping, A. Anguita, A. Bucur, T.C. Cirstea, D. Jacobs, and A. Torge. Improving the implementation of clinical decision support systems, *Engineering in Medicine and Biology Society, 35th Annual International Conference of the IEEE*, (2013), 3214-3217.

[4] A. Lahsasna, R. Noor, R. Zainuddin, A. Bulgiba, Design of a fuzzy-based decision support system for coronary heart disease diagnosis, *Journal of Medical Systems*, **36**(5) (2012), 3293-306.

[5] P. Jensen, L. Jensen,S. Brunak, Mining electronic health records: towards better research applications and clinical care, *Nature Reviews. Genetics*, **13**(6) (2012), 395-405.

[6] A. Sen, A. Banerjee, A. Sinha, M. Bansal, Clinical decision support: Converging toward an integrated architecture. *Journal of Biomedical Informatics*, **45**(5) (2012), 1009 - 1017.

[7] S. H. Liao, P.-H. Chu, P.Y. Hsiao, Data mining techniques and applications: A decade review from 2000 to 2011, *Expert Systems with Applications*, 39(12), (2012), 11303 – 11311.

[8] E.W.T. Ngai, Y. Hu, Y.H. Wong, Y. Chen, X. Sun, The application of data mining techniques in financial fraud detection: A classification framework and an academic review of literature, *Decision Support Systems*, **50**(3) (2011), 559 – 569.

[9] R. Isola, R. Carvalho, A.K. Tripathy, Knowledge discovery in medical systems using differential diagnosis, LAMSTARR & k/NN, *IEEE Transactions on Information Technology in Biomedicine*, **16**(6) (2012), 1287- 1295.

[10] G. Štiglic, S. Kocbek, I. Pernek, P. Kokol, Comprehensive decision tree models in bioinformatics, *PLoS One*, **7**(3) (2012).

[11] H. Jinliang, Y. Caiqing, L. Jiansheng, S. Jianjing, Research on clinical diagnostic models of IPF syndromes in TCM based on dynamic Kohonen network and decision tree, *Intell Sys,* **2** (2010), 107-110.

[12] I. Yoo, P. Alafaireet, M. Marinov, K. Pena-Hernandez, R. Gopidi, J. Chang, L. Hua, Data mining in healthcare and biomedicine, *Journal of Medical Systems*, **36**(4) (2012), 2431-2448.

[13] N. Marín, C. Molina, J. M. Serrano, A. Vila, A complexity guided algorithm for association rule extraction on fuzzy datacubes, *IEEE Tras. on Fuzzy Systems*, **16** (2008), 693-714.

[14] K. Bache, M. Lichman. UCI machine learning repository, http://archive.ics.uci.edu/ml/, 2013.

[15] S. Guillaume, B. Charnomordic, Generating an interpretable family of fuzzy partitions from data, **12**(3) (2004), 324-335.

Cross-Border Challenges in Informatics with a Focus on Disease Surveillance and Utilising Big Data 97
L. Stoicu-Tivadar et al. (Eds.)

doi:10.3233/978-1-61499-389-6-97

The Effect of the Waiting Times on the Patient Pathways for Patients with Suspected Coronary Artery Disease

Ferenc KIRÁLY[a1], István KÓSA[a,b] and István VASSÁNYI[a]

[a]*Medical Informatics R&D Center, University of Pannonia, Veszprém, Hungary*
[b]*Cardiac Rehabilitation Centre of Military Hospital, Balatonfüred, Hungary*

Abstract. The paper describes the investigation of the Hungarian public administrative health databases with the aim to identify hidden correspondences in the patients' evaluation pathways for patients with suspected coronary artery disease (CAD). In our current work we investigated the effect of the waiting times of invasive and non-invasive investigations in the evaluation pathways of patients with suspected CAD. We found a considerable correlation between waiting times and the further course of the patients.

Keywords. Waiting time, Coronary artery disease, CAD, Patient evaluation pathways, Invasive procedure, Non-invasive procedure, Public administrative health databases.

Introduction

There are clinical guidelines describing the optimal evaluation process of patients with suspected coronary artery disease (CAD) in every health care system [1-3], but there is a considerable gap between these guidelines and the clinical practice in most countries [4-5].

Both the financial incentive of patients motivated by maximal return on social security contributions, as well as the defensive nature of decision making by the medical staff drive the service toward the procedure intensive patient pathways, even though such deviations result in some cases in the increase of the patient risk. Since this bias induces also considerable excess resource utilization, the exploration of such deviations has utmost importance for any health financing system. The contextual evaluation of medical decisions is, however, a very hard task, so most health systems rely on the utilization of simple mechanical limits. In the current work, we depict a method for the systematic evaluation of the regional health system, relying on the data of administrative hospital event records and data of the national death register.

[1] Corresponding Author.

Our main goal in the presented work was to investigate if there is any effect of the waiting times for the cardiac imaging investigation on the evolution of patient pathways.

1. Materials and method

We included 488,934 patients (231.683 men and 257.251 women, mean age 54.04±14.20) into our analysis, identified by their pseudo social security number from the depersonalized database of the National Institute for Quality- and Organizational Development in Healthcare and Medicines, Hungary, for whom diagnostic tests such as stress ECG (SECG), stress perfusion single photon emission computed tomography / echocardiography (non-invasive stress investigation, henceforth "NII") or coronary angiography (invasive investigation, henceforth "II"), were performed to assess symptoms suspect for CAD between 01.01.2004 and 31.12.2008. This data set was provided free for research purposes. Survival data were also available from the death registry until 31.12.2009.

Data cleaning, modeling and analysis have been demonstrated in more detail previously [6, 7]. Briefly, we created a coded event list for each patient using the International Classification of Diseases (ICD) codes and International Classification of Procedures in Medicine (ICPM) codes of the source database. We also created a death event from each death case in the death registry. In the second step, we merged coded event sequences into a single real event, based on a set of common sense rules describing our clinical coding practice. Then we selected patients with stable conditions as those having no diagnosis of acute myocardial infarction and having coronary angiography in a direct invasive (DI) way (i.e. there were no previous investigations prior to the invasive investigation procedure) after a 6 month long event-free period. The aim of this selection method was to investigate only whole patient episodes, marked by a long event free period in the event list of the patient.

Since we had access to the postal code (ZIP) of the patients, we performed a spatial analysis of patient pathways. For each patient, we defined her/his primary care provider as the provider of her/his first stress electrocardiography in the observation period. Our ZIP area clustering procedure then identified 136 primary cardiology centers (PCC's) based on care records of patients living in the area supplied dominantly by the centre. For every PCC with more than 100 SECG procedures, the incidence of SECG, NII and II, as well as the waiting times for such investigations after a SECG and the revascularization rate at the time of the first follow-up investigation (RR), were calculated.

2. Results

The average incidence of SECG, NII and II as initial investigation were 427.56± 170.13, 35.3 ± 19.6, and 29.8 ± 11.6, respectively (NII vs. II p=ns). The average waiting times were 47.2 ± 12.2 and 44.9 ± 12.3 days (p=ns) for NII and II, respectively. The RR was 24.5 ± 5.1%. Neither II, nor NII incidence, but both II and NII waiting times correlated with RR ($r = 0.48$, $p < 0.001$, $r = 0.42$, $p = 0.001$, respectively). The correlation between the II waiting times and the RR is shown in Figure 1. The correlation between NII waiting time and RR is shown in Figure 2.

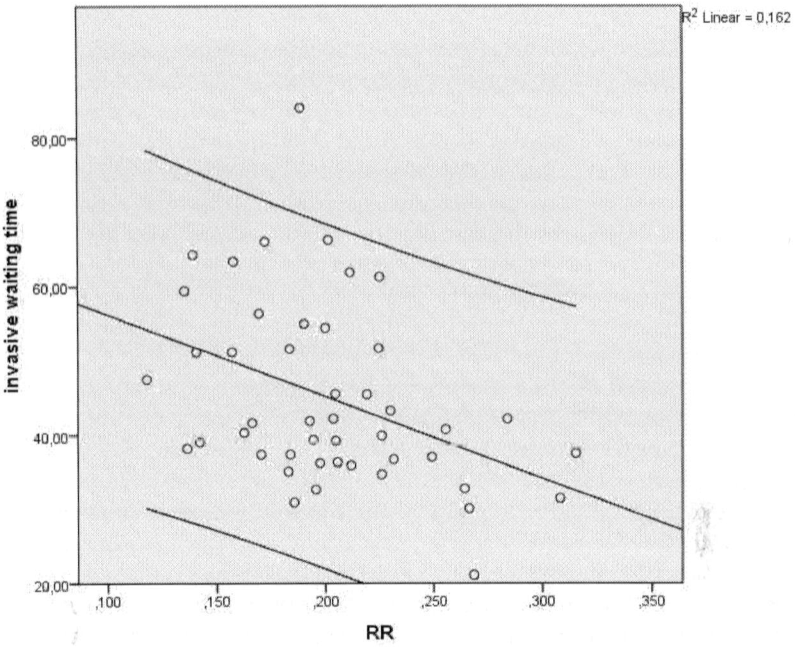

Figure 1. Correlation between II waiting time and RR

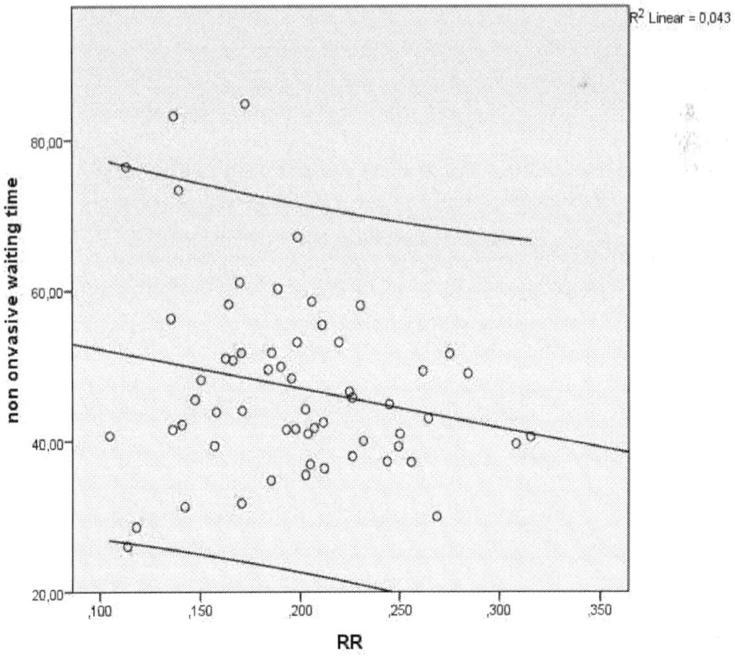

Figure 2. Correlation between NII waiting time and RR

3. Discussion

In the current study, we demonstrated that the length of waiting time correlates with the frequency of revascularisation rate. The heterogeneity of patient selection for invasive investigations is a well known phenomenon. The interpretation of clinical status of the patients is a subjective process, in which the carefulness of the cardiologist, the time she/he spends to evaluation of the complaints of the patients and of course her/his professional mentality are the determinant factors. It is well known that several physicians over-emphasize the benefit of invasive treatment and for this reason, they select more patients for invasive investigation than justified. Earlier we demonstrated that from those areas where the referral rate for invasive coronary angiography as initial investigation is high, patients with relatively lower mortality risk arrive to the catheter laboratory, than from areas with lower direct invasive frequency [7]. Similarly, it was demonstrated that the proximity of such invasive facilities correlates with the mortality risk of stable angina patients referred for direct invasive evaluations [8]. Earlier we have not investigated the effect of this selection bias on the following revascularisation, but it is known that the normalcy rate of referred patient, as well as the revascularisation rate demonstrates considerable regional variations. In a recent work Cotarlan et al. investigated the practice of 76 veteran administration cardiac catheterization labs, and demonstrated that the median proportion of normal coronaries in the lowest quartile was 10.8%, as compared with a median proportion of 19.1% in the second lowest quartile, 23.1% in the second highest quartile, and 30.3% in the highest quartile [9]. Hospitals with lower rates of normal coronaries had higher rates of subsequent revascularization (38.1% vs 33.9% vs 31.5% vs 29.3%, P<.001).

4. Conclusions

Based on this type of assessment we can conclude that the availability of both noninvasive imaging and invasive imaging techniques influences the evolution of patient pathways. Theoretically, the better availability of noninvasive imaging facilities may improve patient selection. In the background of the similar correlation between invasive imaging frequency and following revascularisation frequency, the role of better patient selection also cannot be excluded, but based on our earlier work, demonstrating lower mortality risk in high direct invasive frequency areas, neither a higher frequency of unjustified revascularizations can be excluded. To clarify this question we need further investigations.

The conclusions of the analysis presented in this paper can be exploited in the design of eHealth clinical trials and for the validation tests of prototype e-Health information systems.

Acknowledgements

The work presented was supported by the European Union and co-funded by the European Social Fund, project title: "Telemedicine-focused research activities in the field of Mathematics, Informatics and Medical Sciences", project number: TÁMOP-4.2.2.A-11/1/KONV-2012-0073.

References

[1] K. Fox, M.A.A. Garcia, D. Ardissino, P. Buszman et al., Guidelines on the management of stable angina pectoris: executive summary: The Task Force on the Management of Stable Angina Pectoris of the European Society of Cardiology, *Eur. Heart J*, **27** (2006), 1341–1381.

[2] P. Kolh, W. Wijns, N. Danchin, C. Di Mario et al., Guidelines on myocardial revascularization, *European Journal of Cardio-Thoracic Surgery* **38** (Supplement 1) (2010), S1–S52.

[3] L. Smeeth, J.S. Skinner, J. Ashcroft, H. Hemingway, A. Timmis, NICE clinical guideline: chest pain of recent onset, *Br J Gen Pract* **60** (2010), 607–610.

[4] S. Cook, A. Walker, O. Hügli, M. Togni, B. Meier, Percutaneous coronary interventions in Europe: prevalence, numerical estimates, and projections based on data up to 2004, *Clin Res Cardiol* **96** (2007), 375–382.

[5] W. Maier, M. Abay, S. Cook et al., The 2002 European registry of cardiac catheter interventions, *Int J Cardiol* **113** (2006), 299–304.

[6] I. Kósa, I. Vassányi, A. Nemes, J. Hortobágyi, G. Kozmann, Stress ECG utilization in the evaluation of patients with chest pain: The real practice in Hungary with 10 million inhabitants, *Int J Cardiol* **149** (2011), 137-139.

[7] I. Kósa, A. Nemes, E. Belicza, F. Király, I. Vassányi, Regional differences in the utilisation of coronary angiography as initial investigation for the evaluation of patients with suspected coronary artery disease, *Int J Cardiol* **168** (2013), 5012-5015.

[8] F. Király, I. Vassányi, F. Rárosi, A. Nemes, I. Kósa, A regionális vizsgálati frekvenciák és a viszgálatra kerülők halálozási mutatójának összefüggése koszorúérbetegség gyanujával kivizsgálásra kerülő betegekben. *In: Kosa I, Vassanyi I, editors., Az e-Health kihívásai. A XXVI. Neumann Kollokvium kiadványa, Veszprém: Pannon Egyetem,* (2013), 135–138.

[9] S.M. Bradley, T.M. Maddox, M.A. Stanislawski, C.I. O'Donnell, G.K. Grunwald, T.T. Tsai et al., Normal Coronary Rates for Elective Angiography in the VA Health Care System: Insights from the VA CART Program, *J Am Coll Cardiol*, **63**(5), (2013), 417-426.

Cross-Border Challenges in Informatics with a Focus on Disease Surveillance and Utilising Big Data 103
L. Stoicu-Tivadar et al. (Eds.)

doi:10.3233/978-1-61499-389-6-103

Routine Data for Disease Surveillance in the Undeveloped Region of the OR Tambo District of the Eastern Cape Province

Chrispin KABUYA[a], Graham WRIGHT[a,1], Anthony ODAMA[a] and Don O'MAHONEY[a]
[a] *Health Informatics Team, Walter Sisulu University, South Africa*

Abstract. The research team needed to upsize the solution previously tested so that it could expand the routine data collected via tablet computers. The research team identified the general flow of data within clinics. Data was mainly collected from registers, which were later converted to electronic form and checked for duplication. A database was designed for the collection of demographic data (Patient Master Index), which was aimed at eliminating duplication of patients' data in several registers. Open Data Kit (ODK) Collect was setup on Android tablets for collecting disease related routine data, while ODK Aggregate as the storage and aggregates of data captured by ODK Collect and the Patient Master Index for demographic data, were setup on an Apple Mini Mac server. Data collection is in progress. The expected results include improved data quality, reliability and quick access to summary data. Secondly, instant retrieval of patient demographic details and clinic numbers are included. Thirdly, ability to form standard reporting from the SQL database and lastly exporting data into the TIER.net and DHIS systems via CVS files thus eliminating the need for data capturers are shown.

Keywords. Disease Surveillance, Routine data, Clinic Registers, ODK, Data quality.

Introduction

It is accepted that the value of routine data is its availability, reliability and validity for those who are interested in that data for the purposes of disease surveillance, resource allocation and other applications.

This study is an upsize implementation of the project undertaken by the Walter Sisulu University (WSU) Health Informatics Research Team. The previous study data collection focused on Tuberculosis, while in this study the focus is on various kinds of diseases, which were recorded in the adult section of the Mthakulo Community Health Centre (CHC). This CHC is some 30 minutes travel from Mthatha. It is a rural CHC serving some 100,000 people who live in relative poverty.

Wright and Odama [1] have questioned the validity of data collected using government registers in rural clinics. Furthermore, O'Mahony states that the cost of generating and summarising this data is costing nurses valuable time that could be used for patient care [2].

---

[1] Corresponding Author.

1. Methods

The Research team analysed how routine data were generated, stored and used at clinics prior to designing the data flow. Routine data are recorded in a number of clinic registers across various consultation rooms.

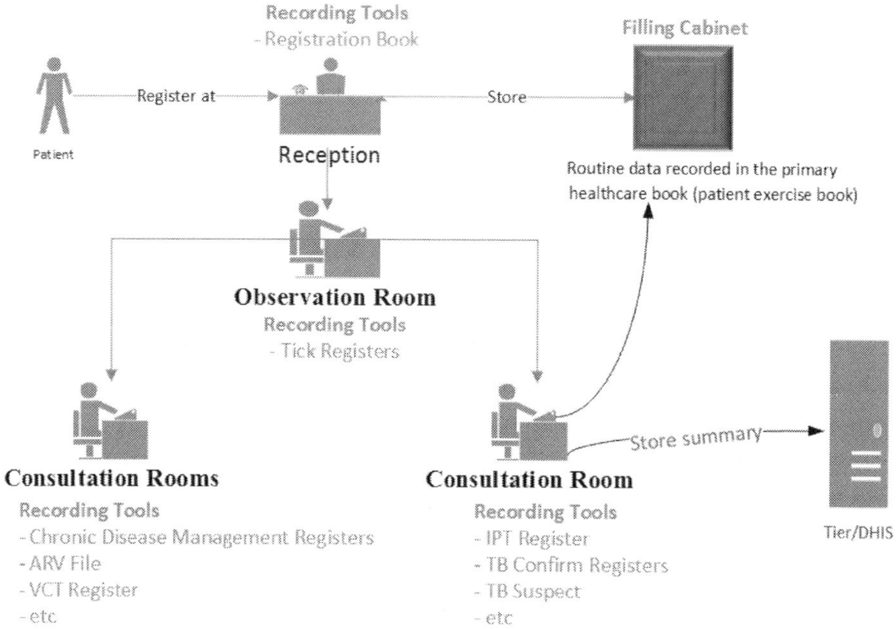

Figure 1. Activity Flow before Introduction of the Solution

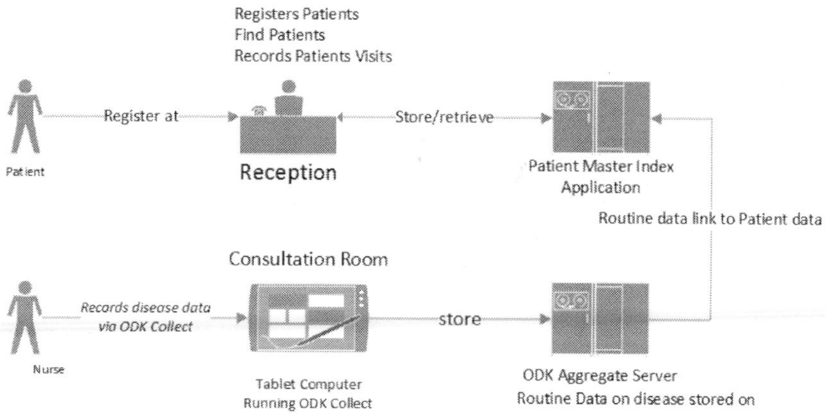

Figure 2. Activity Flow Diagram of Proposed Implementation

The results from the analysis were used to create XForms, which were downloaded to Open Data Kit (ODK) Collect. Processed XForms were used to collect clinical data from the consultation rooms while the Master Patient Index application was used to collect demographic data at the reception.

Having analysed routine data found in registers, the team focused on registers relocated in the adult section of the clinic. The registers included the IPT Register, Chronic Diseases Management Register, HIV Counselling and Testing Register, Chronic Disease and Minor Ailments Register (Tick register) and the TB registers. Data from the registers was separated into clinical data and demographical data. Clinical data was coded into XForms based on registers analysed, while demographical data was coded as HTML5 forms to be used in the Master Patient Index application.

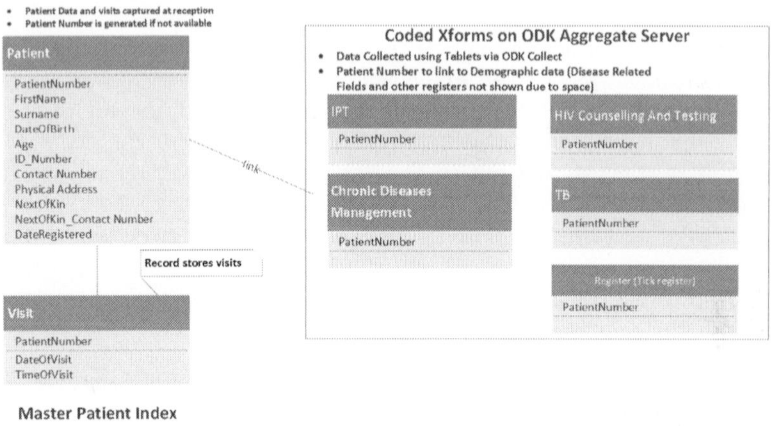

Figure 3 Conceptual Database Schema of the Implementation (without all fields in the ODK Aggregate)

Microsoft Excel was used to design the forms using clinical data collected from registers and then the XLSForm tool was used to convert the forms to XForms so that ODK tools could use them. An ODK Aggregate server was setup on an Apple Mini Server and all XForms created were validated and uploaded to the server. ODK Collect was downloaded from Google Play. It was configured to download XForms from the ODK Aggregate. The forms were tested on tablet computers after they were downloaded from the ODK Aggregate server.

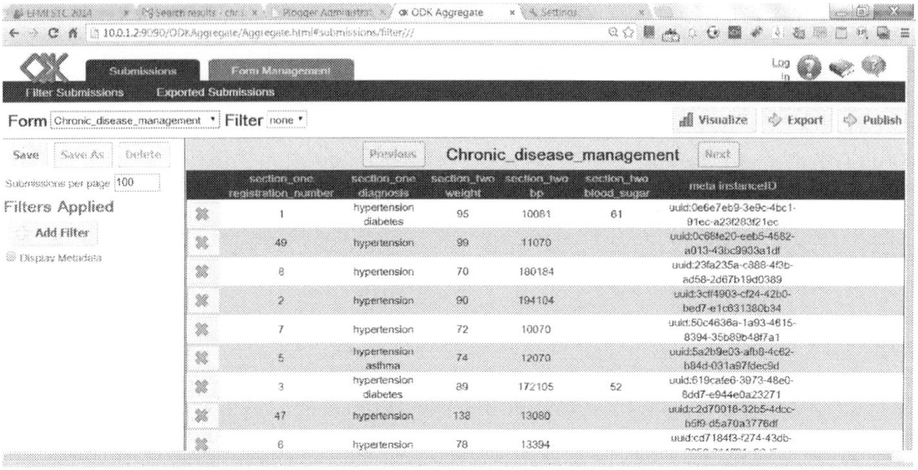

Figure 4. Sample Collected Data on Chronic Disease Management on ODK Aggregate Server

An application (Master Patient Index) to handle routine demographic data was designed using HTML5, Twitter Bootstrap®, Java Enterprise Edition Technologies (Java EE) and open source database MySQL server. Netbeans® Integrated Development Environment (IDE) was used as a developing environment for the application. The Master Patient Index application has the following features: ability to register new patients, to find patients who are already registered, and to record their visits. The application also has statistical reporting features.

In the previous study [3] Google App Engine cloud services were used to host the ODK Aggregate server. However, in this study the team completely avoided using cloud services for security and Internet speed reasons and instead opted for a locally installed tomcat deployment on an Apple Mini server. The research team has computer science skills to manage the deployment, maintenance and support of the tomcat deployment. The Apple Mini server was the best option for the server hardware because of it is ready to run out of the box, easy to install, set up, and manage. Furthermore, its small size makes it ideal for small offices since the clinics we were working in have no dedicated server rooms. Other reasons considered included the ability of the server to automatically backup the hard disk using the Airport Time Capsule, ability to encrypt the hard disk and inbuilt wireless access point which can easily be configured using the Airport Express and Airport Express Extenders.

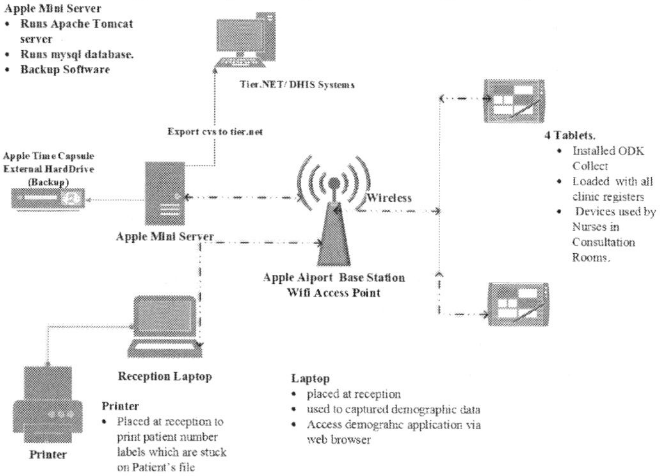

Figure 5. Network Architecture of the Deployment Planning

The Wi-Fi wireless was setup using an inbuilt wireless access point in the Airport Time Capsule and three Airport Express Extenders stations so that the wireless signal was boosted and covered all consultation rooms.

The choice of tablet computers was based on our previous experiences [3]. The team choose tablet computers with only Wi-Fi connection. This was to ensure that nurses were not tempted to connect to 3G networks. The 10.1" tablets running a 4+ version of Android operating system were chosen for this study. Backing up was automated via the Airport Time capsule. Offsite backing up was made easier by both the ODK Aggregate and Master Patient Index applications.

To ensure the smooth operation of this study, members of staff from the reception and the nurses in the consultation rooms were trained to use the ODK Collect and the Master Patient Index application and associated hardware, tablet and laptop computers. Technical and Medical Support was offered by the research team throughout the study.

2. Results and Discussion

As we undertook a pilot project with tablets to collect data we do not foresee any particular problems or issues that we have not addressed in the planning of this project. Early observations indicate that results should include:

- Improved data quality, reliability and quick access to summary & aggregate routine data that could improve disease surveillance in this region. Heunis et al., [4] have also bemoaned the problems of poor data quality. Douglas et al., [5] state that data quality improves the closer it is to the point of capture and if the staff who enter data benefit from the coding. Data is now more reliable since it is captured at the point of care and there is no longer duplication of patient data across registers.
- Instant retrieval of patient demographic details and clinic numbers has drastically reduced waiting times, improved access to statistics on patient visits and improved way to communicate with patients, since all contact details are now readily available throw the Master Patient Index system.
- Ability to form standard reporting from the data stored in the SQL database. Data captured via ODK collect by clinical staff is now available on ODK Aggregate for analysis, export and reporting.
- Exporting of xml instances into the SQL database. Exporting data into the tier.net and DHIS systems via CVS files eliminates the need for data capturers.

3. Conclusion

Given the service delivery problems in the rural clinics and Community Health Centres in the OR Tambo district of the Eastern Cape, South Africa, which include lack of electricity and water supply. Medicines are not delivered in sufficient quantities and there is a lack of medical as well as nursing staff. This study has shown the possibility to design and implement low cost IT solutions to help solve the problems of data capture in rural clinics. The cost of equipment for this project was about 4,000 €.

References

[1] G. Wright, A. Odama, Health Data Ownership and Data Quality: Clinics in the Nyandeni District, Eastern Cape, South Africa, *Engineering Management Research* **1**(2) (2012), 146.

[2] D. O'Mahony, G. Wright, P. Yogeswaran, F. Govere, Knowledge and attitudes of nurses in community health centres about electronic medical records, *Curationis* **37**(1) (2014).

[3] G. Wright, H. J. Betts, J. L. Hernandez Caceres, A. Odama, D. O'Mahony, P. Yogeswaran, F. M. Govere, SLD106 Health Data in Rural Clinics around Mthatha, South Africa: Issues and Possible Solutions, *Informática Salud* **(1)** (2013).

[4] C. Heunis, E. Wouters, G. Kigozi, M. Engelbrecht, Y. Tsibolane, V. Merwe, S. Motlhanke, Accuracy of Tuberculosis Routine Data and Nurses' Views of the TB-HIV Information System in the Free State, South Africa. *Journal of the Association of Nurses in AIDS Care*, **22** (2011), 67-73.

[5] G. P. Douglas, O.J. Gadabu, S. Joukes, S. Mumba, M.V. Mckay, A. Ben-Smith, A. Jahn, E.J. Schouten, Z.L. Lewis, J.J. Van Oosterhout, Using touchscreen electronic medical record systems to support and monitor national scale-up of antiretroviral therapy in Malawi. *PLoS medicine*, **7**(8) (2010), e1000319.

Cross-Border Challenges in Informatics with a Focus on Disease Surveillance and Utilising Big Data 109
L. Stoicu-Tivadar et al. (Eds.)

doi:10.3233/978-1-61499-389-6-109

Usability of HL7 and SNOMED CT Standards in Java Persistence API Environment

Gábor ANTAL[a,1], Ádám Zoltán VÉGH[a] and Vilmos BILICKI[a]
[a] *University of Szeged, Department of Software Engineering*

Abstract. Due to the need for an efficient way of communication between the different stakeholders of healthcare (e.g. doctors, pharmacists, hospitals, patients etc.), the possibility of integrating different healthcare systems occurs. However, during the integration process several problems of heterogeneity might come up, which can turn integration into a difficult task. These problems motivated the development of healthcare information standards. The main goal of the HL7 [1] family of standards is the standardization of communication between clinical systems and the unification of clinical document formats on the structural level. The SNOMED CT [2, 3] standard aims the unification of the healthcare terminology, thus the development of a standard on lexical level. The goal of this article is to introduce the usability of these two standards in Java Persistence API (JPA) [4] environment, and to examine how standard-based system components can be efficiently generated. First, we shortly introduce the structure of the standards, their advantages and disadvantages. Then, we present an architecture design method, which can help to eliminate the possible structural drawbacks of the standards, and makes code generating tools applicable for the automatic production of certain system components.

Keywords. Healthcare information standards, integration, communication, code generation.

Introduction

One of the most important motivations of developing medical information standards was the need for integrated healthcare information systems [5]. Doctors need to communicate with each other, with the hospitals, patients, and pharmacists. Moreover, hospitals also need to keep contact. The connection and communication between local systems can become significantly more efficient if an integrated standard provides the basis of communication. When creating a new healthcare infrastructure it can be more easily integrated with other already existing healthcare systems if it is based on a medical information standard. The main goals of healthcare information standards are speeding up clinical treatments, and improving their quality, reducing costs and risk, improving efficiency, optimizing healthcare workflows, reducing ambiguity and heterogeneity, and improving medical knowledge transferring.

---

[1] Corresponding Author.

The goal of this article is to examine the usability of HL7 and SNOMED CT standards for the efficient development of JPA-based applications and for the automatic generation of certain application components.

1. HL7 Standards

The Health Level 7 (HL7) family of standards is one of the most important representatives of medical information standards. HL7 Inc. created it with the goal of providing a standardized framework for the exchange, integration, sharing and tracking of electronic healthcare information. The two most widely used versions of the standard are HL7 2.x, which was developed in 1989, and HL7 3.x, which was first published is 2005 (it is still under development).

The HL7 Messaging standard aims the support of communication during clinical, financial, administrative and logistic processes with the structural standardization of message contents. HL7 Messaging 2.x defines a simple ASCII-based message format, while version 3.x uses the XML format that offers a clearer structure for clinical messages. Besides integrating message formats, the further goal of HL7 is to standardize the content of clinical documents. For this purpose, the CDA (Clinical Document Architecture [6, 7]) standard was developed, which also defines an XML-based descriptive language for describing the coding, the structure, and the semantics of clinical documents.

For grounding the standards defined by HL7, a model is needed which defines the structure and relations of entities in the healthcare domain. HL7 uses a hierarchic approach to develop this model. On the top of the model hierarchy, we find the RIM (Reference Information Model [8]) model, which describes the structure of clinical and administrative data found in HL7 messages and documents, with their semantic and lexical relationships. The RIM models the healthcare domain with general entities such as patients, devices, observations, documents and employees. The MIM (Message Information Model) models are derived from the RIM. They cover some specific segments within the healthcare domain, e.g. healthcare treatments, clinical decision support, laboratory data, pharmacy, clinical data management, scheduling, finance, tools of therapy.

2. The SNOMED CT Standard

The other important representative of healthcare information standards is the SNOMED CT (Systematized NOmenclature of MEDicine Clinical Terms) standard, which was officially published in January 2002. Its goal is to collect and integrate the elements of healthcare terminology in order to eliminate the problems arising from the linguistic and dialectic differences, and to integrate the terms used in clinical documents and reports. The areas covered by the standard include clinical events, symptoms, diagnoses, processes, tools, and medicines.

The key element of the standard is the concept. It defines a clinical term, and has a unique identification code and a text description. Between the concepts, different relations might be defined. Moreover, each concept has different names: a full name, which is unique considering the whole standard; a preferred name, which is given by the experts of the domain for the unified expression of the concept; and zero or more synonyms referring to the given concept. SNOMED CT can be regarded as an ontology-based multilingual dictionary of synonyms, a class hierarchy beyond the terminology of the healthcare domain. It defines several relations between the classes, e.g. inheritance ("is a") relation, cause and effect ("causative agent") relation, and the relation between synonyms [9].

3. Usability of Standards in JPA Environment

The fundamental goal during the development of a standardized JPA-based application is that the standard that has been used as the base of the system shall define a structure from which the data-representing entities and their relations can be prepared. That means that certain elements of the standard have to be applicable for the preparation of the application's domain model. The domain model hierarchy defined by HL7 provides a general model with significant expert background over the healthcare domain, which can be used in any healthcare context. On the other hand, the standard is quite extensive and covers lots of segments, therefore the models can be difficult to overview and it is hard to find a partial model to a selected segment. SNOMED CT is standardizing the concepts used in the field of medical information technology. However the standard covers only lexical issues, it does not contain structural descriptions therefore it does not define a classic domain model. As a result, between the two presented standards only HL7 can be directly applied to the definitions of the data structures to be stored.

The SNOMED CT, since it is a lexical standard, is not capable for definition of data storage structures. Nevertheless, the domain models of HL7 are too general, and the concepts related to specific segments are being defined with the general HL7 structures, extended with identifiers, which are defining the specific type (for example, the "Systolic blood pressure" measurement data is stored in the general Observation entity, with the corresponding measurement data type code). One of the most important code sets for the specializing identifiers are supplied by the SNOMED CT concept codes. Since the SNOMED CT is functioning also as a multilingual synonym dictionary, it can be used for the standardization of the phrases displayed on the user interfaces of applications. At this time, the label keys referred on the user interfaces are pointing to SNOMED CT codes, through which the name of the concept with the given code can be reached in all the languages supported by the standard, assisting the standardized translation of the application.

4. Development of HL7-based Telemedicine Applications

During the study of the usability of standards, a problem occurred related to the development of a HL7-based ECG measurement data storing and visualizing application. The HL7 recommendation used for the ECG measurements is the HL7 aECG (Annotated ECG [10]) standard, which defines the structure and format of HL7 messages and CDA documents that contains the ECG measurement data. An important characteristic of HL7 aECG is that it defines an exceptionally extensive and general model even for the relatively small domain of the ECG measurements. Therefore during the planning of the application's domain model a minimal partial model of the

HL7 aECG domain model has been defined, which includes the necessary elements for the standardized modeling, and are sufficient for the data modeling defined by the task.

The development of the application was assisted by an internally developed code generating tool, which could automatically generate the DAO (Data Access Object) and business logic layers as well as the user interfaces based on the JPA entities of the application. The selected partial model defines a deep tree structure in which the relevant data for the users (e.g. doctor's data, patient's data, measurement results, data of measurement device etc.) can be found in the leaves of the tree. By generating the prototype of the application from this model, we get user interfaces fitting to the complex domain model structure that are difficult to use. Therefore, we need a solution in which the code generating tool is applicable and the generated user interfaces are usable, but in the meantime the data is being stored in a structure according to the HL7 standard.

The solution for the problem was the implementation of a middle entity layer and a middle DAO layer above the standardized entities and DAO layer. The layers of the modified system architecture can be seen in Figure 1.

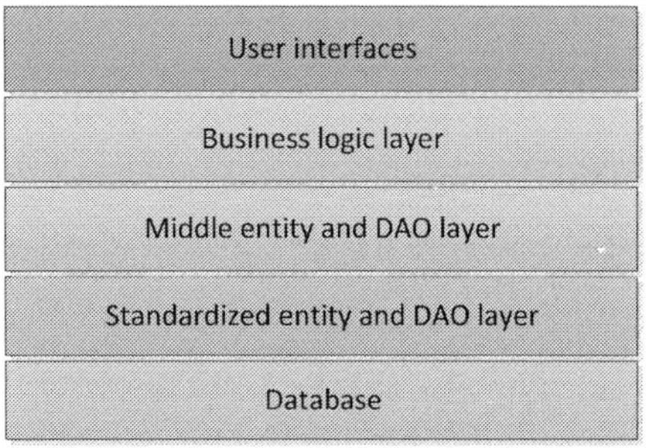

Figure 1. Layers of the modified system architecture

The middle entity layer aims the realization of a domain model, which is more similar to the structure of the data to be presented on the user interfaces. If we generate the application from the middle layer entities instead of the standardized entities then the generated user interfaces will have simpler structures and will be easier to use. As a result the middle layer entities will be displayed on the user interfaces. However, since the data storage is being done according to the standardized entities there is a need for conversion between the two entity layers. The middle DAO layer, which has two major functions, will implement this. The middle DAO layer major functions are building middle layer entities from entities returned by standardized DAO queries, and conversion of middle layer entities built on user interfaces into standardized entities that can be stored. The middle DAO layer has to be prepared manually following the definition of the mapping between the two entity layers. Therefore, the methods of the middle layer DAO will be called from the business logic layer.

5. Conclusions

The structure and importance of the two most notable health information technology standards: HL7 and SNOMED CT is presented here. While HL7 aims the structural standardization of the healthcare domain, SNOMED CT unifies the healthcare terminology lexically. Only HL7 can be used for definition of data storage structures, but the latter one can be adapted for the specialization of the general HL7 entities, as well as the standardized multilingual translations of the healthcare applications' user interfaces. We also presented how the telemedicine applications can be generated based on the HL7 standard with the introduction of middle layer and DAO layer entities above the standardized entities, eliminating the complexity of HL7 domain models.

We used the discussed methodology in the development of an HL7 aECG standard-based ECG data collector application. Our code generation toolkit simplified the implementation of the system significantly, because we have to concentrate only on the data to be visualized on the user interfaces, and the conversion between the standardized entities and visualized middle layer entities. The implementation of the entity conversion is manual now, but we would like to support it with a graphical entity transformation toolkit in the future.

The standard-based development methodology discussed in this paper can be also used in case of other medical information standards, which have well defined domain models to describe the entities of the medical domain, e.g., CEN/ISO 13606 [11].

Acknowledgements

The publication is supported by the European Union and co-funded by the European Social Fund. Project title: "Telemedicine-focused research activities on the field of Mathematics, Informatics and Medical sciences". Project number: TÁMOP-4.2.2.A-11/1/KONV-2012-0073

References

[1] Health Level Seven International – Homepage, http://www.hl7.org/. [Accessed on 16 December 2013].
[2] SNOMED CT, http://www.ihtsdo.org/snomed-ct/. [Accessed on 16 December 2013].
[3] K. Donnelly, SNOMED-CT: The advanced terminology and coding system for eHealth, *Med. Care N.a 3*, **121** (2006), 279-290.
[4] Java Persistence API, http://www.oracle.com/technetwork/java/javaee/tech/persistence-jsp-140049.html. [Accessed on 4 December 2013].
[5] W. E. Hammond, J. J. Cimino, Standards in medical informatics, *Medical Informatics,Computer Applications in Health Care and Biomedicine*, Springer, 2001, 226–250.
[6] HL7 CDA-HL7 Clinical Document Architecture, http://www.hl7.com.au/CDA.htm. [Accessed on 4 December 2013].
[7] R. H. Dolin, L. Alschuler, C. Beebe, P. V. Biron, S. L. Boyer, D. Essin, E. Kimber, T. Lincoln, J. E. Mattison, The HL7 clinical document architecture, *J. Am. Med. Inform. Assoc.*, **8** (2001), 552-569.
[8] Reference Information Model (RIM) Downloads, http://www.hl7.org/implement/standards/rim.cfm. [Accessed on 4 December 2013].
[9] SNOMED CT® User Guide, International Health Terminology Standards Development Organisation, July 2013.
[10] HL7 Standards Product Brief - HL7 Version 3 Standard: Implementation Guide; Annotated ECG (aECG), http://www.hl7.org/implement/standards/product_brief.cfm?product_id=102. [Accessed on 4 December 2013].
[11] The CEN/ISO 13606 Association site, http://www.en13606.org/. [Accessed on 6 March, 2014].

L. Stoicu-Tivadar et al. (Eds.)

doi:10.3233/978-1-61499-389-6-115

New Study Program: Interdisciplinary Postgraduate Specialist Study in Medical Informatics

Mira HERCIGONJA-SZEKERES[a,1], Diana ŠIMIĆ[b], Jadranka BOŽIKOV[c], and Petra VONDRA[b]
[a]*Hrvatsko Zagorje Polytechnic, Krapina, Croatia*
[b] *University of Zagreb, Faculty of Organization and Informatics, Varaždin, Croatia*
[c] *University of Zagreb, School of Medicine, Andrija Štampar School of Public Health, Zagreb, Croatia*

Abstract. Paper presents an overview of the EU funded Project of Curriculum Development for Interdisciplinary Postgraduate Specialist Study in Medical Informatics named MEDINFO to be introduced in Croatia. The target group for the program is formed by professionals in any of the areas of medicine, IT professionals working on applications of IT for health and researchers and teachers in medical informatics. In addition to Croatian students, the program will also provide opportunity for enrolling students from a wider region of Southeast Europe. Project partners are two faculties of the University of Zagreb - Faculty of Organization and Informatics from Varaždin and School of Medicine, Andrija Štampar School of Public Health from Zagreb with the Croatian Society for Medical Informatics, Croatian Chamber of Economy, and Ericsson Nikola Tesla Company as associates.

Keywords: Postgraduate Specialist Study, Medical Informatics, Curriculum

Introduction

The overall objective of the project is to contribute to the development and implementation of the Croatian Qualification Framework through development of a new qualification standard for university specialist in medical informatics. The development of a new postgraduate specialist study program is based on learning outcomes and the proper analysis of student workload and ECTS (European Credit Transfer and Accumulation System).

Specifically, the qualification standard will provide prospective employers (in e.g. health service, IT, public administration, and education sectors) with a well defined framework of knowledge, skills and competences that will improve all aspects of human resource management (needs analysis, recruitment, skills gap analysis, training and development). When the new study program becomes available, health care institutions will benefit from engaging skilled employees, thus increasing capacity to implement sophisticated health information systems. IT sector will benefit from access to skilled workers with complementary skills and competences necessary for implementation of IT solutions in health sector, but also from increased capacity of the health sector market to

[1] Corresponding Author.

absorb their products and services. Institutes of public health and national and local authorities responsible for health system will also benefit from both the access to skilled workforce and the health care institutions' increased capacity to implement the national eHealth program. Medical informatics lecturers/teachers with appropriate knowledge and skills can improve medical informatics education at different levels of medical/health education. Finally, the citizens will benefit from the increase in quality and efficiency of health care system due to the successful implementation of eHealth projects.

1. Description of the Project

1.1. Target groups

The target group for the new postgraduate specialist programme in medical informatics is formed by professionals in any of the areas of medicine: nursing, health care management, dentistry, pharmacy, public health, health record administration, informatics/computer science and others who work in health sector, in public authorities responsible for health, and in IT sector designing and developing ICT solutions for health. Due to the introduction of the health information systems, they have a need to attain additional specific skills and competences in medical informatics. Most health professionals who attained their degree at Croatian universities have had a single course in medical informatics during their study program. Most IT professionals who attained their degree at Croatian universities had no exposure to health specific issues in ICTs. Additionally, professionals from other disciplines like mathematics, physics, biology etc. often provide support for informatics in health care institutions. Implementation of health information systems requires that they take part in reengineering the processes in health service institutions, modeling, defining and capturing health data, searching and using different sources of information in decision making, defining business and functional requirements for procurement of information and communication equipment and solutions etc.

Another target group is formed by researchers and teachers in medical informatics. The project will contribute to the development of capacity for implementation of student centered learning and recognition of prior learning through the training of academic staff of participating institutions and targeted study visits to European institutions of higher education with recognized and successful study programs in health/medical (bio)informatics. However, there is a lack of capacity for developing methodology for assessment and recognition of non-formal and in-formal prior learning. The proposed life-long-learning program targets working population who have attained some skills and competences through on-the-job training, work experience or self-learning. It will provide more value to students and their employers if it includes well defined procedures and criteria for assessing and recognizing prior learning, thus focusing on filling the skills gap and increasing effectiveness and efficiency of delivery for both students and their employers. During the implementation of the Bologna process and drafting new study programs Faculty of Organization and Informatics has developed and implemented an application for describing and managing entry competences, prerequisites and learning outcomes of a study program, modules and courses that is used for developing and managing currently offered curricula. Defining the functional requirements and designing the upgrade of the application to include prior learning (formal, in-formal and non-formal) will require practical implementation of knowledge attained through the training. Upgraded and improved application will enable more efficient development and management of the new curriculum, ascertaining consistency of different study paths.

While our primary target is Croatian workforce, the program will also provide opportunity for enrolling students from a wider region of Southeast Europe. Now no similar graduate level program is available in the region. For students from countries in the region Croatian language does not pose a barrier, and for others the program will initially provide a limited offer of study paths in English, with plan to develop all courses / modules in English within two years of the beginning of the program implementation.

1.2. Project Partners and Associates

Faculty of Organization and Informatics (FOI) has extensive experience with managing and participating in EU funded projects, and in particular projects related to defining learning outcomes, training needs assessment and development of study programs. FOI also has strong research, teaching and practice track record in organization, information systems, and e-learning. FOI has participated in a large number of Tempus projects that supported implementation of Bologna process, introduced new student centered study programs and developed capacity for quality assessment.

School of Medicine, Andrija Štampar School of Public Health (ŠNZ) has a strong track record of research, teaching and practice of health/medical informatics. Within its organizational structure there is a Department of Medical Statistics, Epidemiology and Medical Informatics with a Division for Medical Informatics. In the period from 1987 to 1998 ŠNZ offered a postgraduate scientific master program in Health Information System leading to the Master of Science degree.

Croatian Society for Medical Informatics (CSMI) was established in 1989. Since 1992 it is a member of the European Federation for Medical Informatics (EFMI) and the International Medical Informatics Association (IMIA). Their membership comprises health and ICT professional, as well as researchers, representatives of health care and public health institutions and private sector providers of ICT equipment and solutions. Biannual, 10th conference Medical Informatics 2011 held in Varaždin and co-organized by FOI and ŠNZ was an opportunity for discussion of needs for continuing education in medical informatics with all stakeholders.

The Croatian Chamber of Economy (CCE) is an independent professional and business organisation of all legal entities engaging in business. It was established in 1852, organised in the European tradition and on the so-called continental model of Austrian and German chambers with compulsory membership. Every company registered with the Commercial Court is a member of the Chamber. CCE, as a representative of employers, has a strong interest in development of the Croatian Qualification Framework and qualification standards.

Ericsson Nikola Tesla (ENT) is the provider of the national Healthcare Networking Information System that implements Electronic Healthcare Records, Electronic Patient Records, Healthcare Resources Records and Messaging and business processes. Users in healthcare and administration, as well as developers of new health information systems have to know how to interact with this infrastructure. Through implementation and maintenance of the system, ENT has gained the first-hand experience and had to address lack of skills and competences in the health sector. ENT employs research staff who will take part in developing and implementing specific parts of the curriculum, and they can help in dissemination through their extensive contact network.

1.3. Project organization

The project (The duration of the action will be 18 months.) will be organized in eight work-packages (WP) with 21 activities:

- WP-01 Needs Analysis: Systematic literature review; Development of a questionnaire and brainstorming framework and data collection; Data analysis and drafting the Needs Assessment Report.
- WP-02 Building staff capacity: Trainings; Study visits.
- WP-03 Logistics: Improving and updating the existing software; Installation and maintenance of software and hardware; Public procurement and subcontracting.
- WP-04 Development of the study program and the qualification standard of postgraduate specialist in medical informatics: Drafting the study program; Drafting the guidelines for recognition of prior learning; Drafting the documents on quality assurance; Drafting the qualification standard; Workshop and consultations with stakeholders on draft documents.
- WP-05 Developing course content, teaching and e-Learning materials: Development of course content; Development of teaching and e-Learning materials.
- WP-06 Pilot implementation: Piloting and evaluating the study program.
- WP-07 Dissemination: Establishing a project web site; Establishing an online collaboration space; Presenting project results at professional and research conferences; Publishing a book.
- WP-08 Project management.

2. Conclusion remarks

Introduction of qualification standard of medical informatics specialist and the study program in medical informatics with well-defined core competencies will help human resource management in health care, ICT and health administration sectors, increase the capacity of health care organizations to design, develop, implement and use ICT solutions, and consequently increase health care quality, improve patient safety and reduce costs.

Project partners and associates will use the following channels for dissemination: Workshops and conferences, Web site and special web services (FAQ, discussion forum, mailing list, electronic newsletter, blog, collaboration tool etc.), Press releases, radio, TV, promotional activities in local and regional community, Promotional materials (Project leaflet and brochure, banner), Word of mouth (by experts in medical informatics), Book compiling project methodology, training materials and results.

Dissemination plan is scheduled over three phases that roughly cover 6 months each. The first phase comprises activities focusing on building partners' capacity for developing the study program and qualification standard. Dissemination activities planned for this phase include the kick-off meeting, Project Steering Committee meetings, and publishing documents on the project collaboration site targeting the project consortium with the purpose of internal dissemination and coordination; press release(s) targeting media and general public with a purpose of announcing the EU support; project leaflet and brochure, web site and special web services targeting stakeholders and general public with the purpose of awareness raising; workshops with stakeholders with the purpose of awareness raising and feedback; and conference presentations targeting professionals and academics in medical informatics and their potential employers with the purpose of awareness raising and feedback.

The second phase covers drafting the main documents. Dissemination activities planned for this phase include the Project Steering Committee meetings and publishing documents on the project collaboration site targeting the project consortium with the purpose of internal dissemination and coordination; project reports, web site and special web services targeting stakeholders and general public with the purpose of providing information on project status and the awareness raising; workshops with stakeholders with the purpose of awareness raising and feedback; and conference presentations targeting professionals and academics in medical informatics and their potential employers with the purpose of awareness raising and feedback.

The third phase involves piloting and finalization of the project. Dissemination activities planned for this phase include the Project Steering Committee meetings and publishing documents on the project collaboration site targeting the project consortium with the purpose of internal dissemination and coordination; project reports, web site and special web services targeting stakeholders and general public with the purpose of providing information on project status and the awareness raising; conference presentations targeting professionals and academics in medical informatics and their potential employers with the purpose of awareness raising and feedback; the book and a press release targeting general public, stakeholders and wider academic community with the purpose of informing about the project results and promoting their reuse.

Both partners FOI and ŠNZ are determined to certify the program as a joint study program, and are open to participation of other institutions and experts in further development, maintenance and implementation of the qualification standard and the study program.

Acknowledgement

This project is funded by the European Union through the national IPA BGUE 04 06 – Human Resources Development, under the grant number IPA4.1.3.1.06.01.c12.

References

[1] http://www.foi.unizg.hr/eng [visited 2/1/2014]
[2] http://www.mef.unizg.hr/eng/ [visited 2/1/2014]
[3] http://www.hdmi.hr/ [visited 2/1/2014]
[4] http://en.hgk.hr/ [visited 2/1/2014]
[5] http://www.ericsson.hr/homepage [visited 2/1/2014]
[6] http://www.amzh.hr/news%20and%20events.html [visited 2/1/2014]
[7] A. Hasman, J. Mantas, IMIA Accreditation of Health Informatics Programs, *Healthc Inform Res.* **19**(3) (2013), 154-161.
[8] J. Mantas, E. Ammenwerth, G. Demiris, A. Hasman, R. Haux, W. Hersh, E. Hovenga, K.C. Lun, H. Marin, F. Martin-Sanchez, G. Wright, Recommendations of the International Medical Informatics Association (IMIA) on Education in Biomedical and Health Informatics. First Revision, *Methods Inf Med.* **49**(2) 2010, 105-120.
[9] http://www.imia-medinfo.org/new2/node/8 [visited 2/1/2014]
[10] http://ec.europa.eu/europeaid/work/visibility/documents/communication_and_visibility_manual_en.pdf [visited 2/1/2014]
[11] http://ec.europa.eu/budget/execution/legal_entities_fr.htm [visited 2/1/2014]

Posters

L. Stoicu-Tivadar et al. (Eds.)

doi:10.3233/978-1-61499-389-6-123

Evaluating Study for a Multiuser Oriented Medical Data Visualization Method

Georgy KOPANITSA[a,b]
[a] *Institute Cybernetic Center, Tomsk Polytechnic University, Lenina 30, Tomsk, Russia*
[b] *Tomsk State University for Architecture and Building, Tomsk, Russia*

Keywords. Evaluation, Visualization, Archetype

Introduction

Evaluation of EHR systems supports implementation and provides feedback to developers. Evaluation tests approach feasibility and methods according to specified goals. Main evaluation criteria are functionality, acceptability, usefulness and usability, but they may vary. The chosen evaluation approach is based on the Guideline for Good Evaluation Practice in Health Informatics (GEP-III). The guidelines provide framework for the evaluation of EHR systems but do not specify the concrete evaluation methods.

1. Methods

The scheme evaluates standard based medical data visualization method developed within the ByMedConnect (BMC) project in a hospital environment. Method is based on a visual medical concept (VMC) that complements the archetype layer of ISO 13606.

2. Results

After the recruitment process the evaluation study, included doctors and patients divided into two groups. For doctors the criteria was the experience with Avrora EHR and for patients the age. The evaluators were independent people with a medical background, trained and divided into groups; working only with doctors or only with patients.

3. Discussion

Evaluation study demonstrates the efficiency of the system for both doctors and patients. It decreases time working with EHR and provides efficient data representation for different user groups. Solution gives users a better control on the system by providing efficient modelling facilities, being the main motivating factor to use the system. The rate of data misinterpretations is very low in comparison with paper-based processes.

Cross-Border Challenges in Informatics with a Focus on Disease Surveillance and Utilising Big Data 125
L. Stoicu-Tivadar et al. (Eds.)

doi:10.3233/978-1-61499-389-6-125

Mobile Learning Readiness of Nursing Students

Neşe ZAYİM[a,1] and Deniz ÖZEL[a]
[a]*Akdeniz University, Turkey*

Keywords. Mobile learning, Nursing, Readiness.

Introduction

Mobile learning use and acceptance varies based on both personal and technological factors. Financial limitations, technology proficiency level, age are suggested personal factors, which enhance mobile learning interest. Self-directed learning abilities are significant indicators of readiness for mobile learning. Definitive analyses of potential users and readiness of learning environments contributes significantly to the success of mobile learning application efforts. This study is to determine readiness, attitudes, and preferences of nursing students with respect to mobile learning environments.

1. Methods

A survey has been used to investigate the preferences and opinions of nursing students in relation to mobile learning. The survey was distributed to a total of 436 students who were asked to participate voluntarily. The response rate of students was 89% (387/436).

2. Results

Participants are 62.6% female and 37.4% male with a mean age of 20.57 ± 1.81. In terms of class distribution, the majority is freshmen level and the minority is fourth year seniors. Half of survey participants consider themselves good or very good computer users. In terms of device ownership, order of descending frequency is mobile phones, laptops, and smart phones. Nearly 60% of students have indicated ownership of two or more devices.

3. Discussion

Technology use alone is not sufficient for success in learning. Important factors such as technological readiness, attitudes, and adoption by users should also be taken into consideration. Through assessments of readiness, skills, weaknesses or strengths as well as threats and opportunities, and requirements can be identified.

[1] Corresponding Author.

Cross-Border Challenges in Informatics with a Focus on Disease Surveillance and Utilising Big Data 127
L. Stoicu-Tivadar et al. (Eds.)

doi:10.3233/978-1-61499-389-6-127

Application of Electronic Health Record System for Teaching Medical Students

Sergey KARAS[a,1], Eduard MERKER[b], Irina KORNEVA[b], Alexey PONOMAREV[b] and Georgy KOPANITSA[b,c,d]
[a] *Siberian State Medical University, Lenina 30, Tomsk, Russia*
[b] *UMSSoft, Gagarina 11/1, Tomsk Russia*
[c] *Institute Cybernetic Center, Tomsk Polytechnic University, Tomsk, Russia*
[d] *Tomsk State University for Architecture and Building, Tomsk, Russia*

Keywords. Learning Electronic Health Record, UML, Medical Education

Introduction

Despite IT development of Russian healthcare, the level of IT competence of physicians remains low. This creates a sustainable obstacle for the introduction of modern IT technologies to the healthcare system. A specific learning EHR (LEHR) can improve clinical and IT competences of medical students. This can be achieved by integration of an EHR to the programs of all clinical subjects combining clinical and IT knowledge.

1. Methods

The analysis of educational programs showed a high potential of their implementation in the LEHR due to well-structured and high formalization. The next step is engineering of expert knowledge applying active cognitive methods with further anonymized discussion.

2. Results

Interaction of an end-user with LEHR is Web-based and performed through a thin client. This is achieved via three level architecture in cooperation with Role Based Access Control (RBAC), which provide service accessibility, roles distinctions, and efficient data access. We use MSSQL 2012 along with Application Request Routing (ARR).

3. Discussion

The future development of LEHR for other clinical subjects will be based on the technical specification that being developed. The introduction of the LEHR into the educational process will support adoption of IT by the medical students in Russia.

---

[1] Corresponding Author.

L. Stoicu-Tivadar et al. (Eds.)

doi:10.3233/978-1-61499-389-6-129

Proof of Concept Using Tablet Computers to Survey TB

Anthony ODAMA[a], Graham WRIGHT[a,1], Chrispin KABUYA[a] and Don O'MAHONY[a]
[a]*Health Informatics Team, Walter Sisulu University, South Africa*

Keywords. Survey, Routine Data, Tablet Computer, Disease Surveillance

Introduction

This study took place in a rural clinic in the OR Tambo district of the Eastern Cape province in SA. It explored two distinct issues: First, attitudes of nurses to technology, given that a previous study showed lack of knowledge and skill in using computers and second, feasibility of using ODK as a survey instrument to collect TB data at the clinic.

1. Methods

Two members of the health informatics team interviewed all the nurses before and after we tried out tablets using a standard set of questions. The main thrust of this paper is the second part of the project, which involves introducing tablet computers, most specifically open source software, Open Data Kit (ODK).

2. Results

We collected valid information regarding patient status using x-forms, and in addition received positive feedback from the nurses on the ease of use of the programme (ODK).

3. Discussion

This project was undertaken as a "proof of concept" study, validated the hypothesis that tablet computers could be used for data collection, as a majority of the nurses were familiar with mobile telephones, and found it easy to learn to use the tablet. This study allowed us to formulate a full-blown research project, which is the subject of the paper entitled: Routine data for Disease surveillance in the undeveloped region of the OR Tambo District of the Eastern Cape province in South Africa.

[1] Corresponding Author.

L. Stoicu-Tivadar et al. (Eds.)

Subject Index

L. Stoicu-Tivadar et al. (Eds.)

Author Index